Royal Society of Medicine

International Congress and Symposium Series

Editor-in-Chief: H.-J. C. L'Etang

Number 73

Nocturnal Asthma

Proceedings of a meeting sponsored by Napp Laboratories at the Royal Society of Medicine, London, on 17th February 1984

Royal Society of Medicine

International Congress and Symposium Series

Number 73

Nocturnal Asthma

Edited by
P. J. BARNES AND J. LEVY

1984

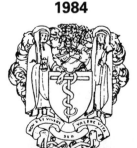

Published by
THE ROYAL SOCIETY OF MEDICINE
1 Wimpole Street, London

ROYAL SOCIETY OF MEDICINE
1 Wimpole Street, London W1M 8AE

Distributed by
OXFORD UNIVERSITY PRESS
Walton Street, Oxford OX2 6DP

London   New York   Toronto
Delhi   Bombay   Calcutta   Madras   Karachi
Kuala Lumpur   Singapore   Hong Kong   Tokyo
Nairobi   Dar es Salaam   Cape Town
Melbourne   Auckland

and associated companies in
Beirut   Berlin   Ibadan   Mexico City   Nicosia

Oxford is a trade mark of Oxford University Press

Copyright © 1984 by

ROYAL SOCIETY OF MEDICINE

The sponsors of this Symposium are responsible for both the scientific and literary content of this publication. The views expressed are not necessarily those of the Royal Society of Medicine. Distribution has been in accordance with the wishes of the sponsors but a copy is available to any Fellow of the Society at a privileged price.

British Library Cataloguing in Publication Data.

Nocturnal asthma.—(Royal Society of Medicine
  international congress and symposium series,
  ISSN 0142-2367; no. 73)
  1. Asthma
  I. Barnes, P.J.   II. Levy, J.   III. Series
  616.2'38   RC591

  ISBN 0-19-922011-5

Printed in Great Britain at the University Press, Oxford

Contributors

P. J. Barnes

Department of Medicine, Hammersmith Hospital and Royal Postgraduate Medical School, London, UK

T. J. Clark

Guy's Hospital, London, UK

G. M. Cochrane

New Cross and Guy's Hospital, London, UK

N. J. Douglas

Edinburgh Royal Infirmary, Edinburgh, Scotland

A. Fairfax

Department of Thoracic Medicine, Stafford General Infirmary, Stafford, UK

D. C. Flenley

Department of Respiratory Medicine, University of Edinburgh, City Hospital Edinburgh, Scotland

A. P. Greening

City Hospital, Edinburgh, Scotland

M. R. Hetzel

Whittington and University College Hospitals, London, UK

D. Minors

Department of Physiology, University of Manchester, Manchester, UK

A. Newman-Taylor

Brompton Hospital, London, UK

D. Pavia

Department of Thoracic Medicine, Royal Free Hospital and School of Medicine, London, UK

M. Turner-Warwick

Brompton Hospital, London, UK

Contents

Introduction

P.J. BARNES

Department of Medicine, Hammersmith Hospital, London W12, UK.

D.C. FLENLEY

Department of Respiratory Medicine, University of Edinburgh, City Hospital, Edinburgh, UK.

Worsening of asthma at night and in the early morning has been recognized since the first known descriptions of the disease. Dr John Floyer (1698), a London physician, vividly described his own attacks of asthma, which came on exclusively at night over seven years. He wrote, 'I have often observed the fit always to happen after sleep in the night, when nerves are filled with the windy spirits and the heat of the bed has rarified the spirits and humours.' The frequency of asthma attacks at night has long been recognized, but it is only recently that nocturnal asthma has been carefully studied and its mechanisms investigated. The study of wheezing at night has been greatly aided by simple objective measurements of airway obstruction, such as the peak expiratory flow (PEF). Such studies have revealed that an 'early morning dip' in PEF is a common occurrence in asthma and have uncovered the presence of asthma in patients who have no evidence of airway obstruction during the day, and who have often remained undiagnosed (Turner-Warwick 1977). The clinical importance of nocturnal asthma is emphasized by the observation that in most series there has been an excess of sudden death and episodes of ventilatory arrest in asthmatics at night and in the early hours of the morning. (*Lancet* 1983).

Dr Thomas Willis, who wrote the definitive text on treatment in the seventeenth century (Willis 1679), believed that wheezing at night could be explained by overheating of the blood by the bedclothes, which caused 'more plentiful sucking of air'. Since then many possible causes for nocturnal asthma have been proposed, but it is only recently that the underlying mechanisms have become clearer (Hetzel 1981; Barnes 1984). Understanding the causes of nocturnal asthma is important if effective therapy is to be given. It may prove surprisingly difficult to treat nocturnal symptoms, which often persist when asthma is well controlled during the day. Indeed, controlling nocturnal symptoms without further disturbing the quality of sleep in asthmatic patients remains one of the most important challenges in the management of asthma today.

For these reasons there has recently been a great deal of interest in nocturnal asthma. The purpose of this symposium is to discuss what is known of underlying mechanisms, then to consider currently available treatment for this troublesome condition. Armed with this information a logical approach to treatment can be followed and the requirements for effective therapy clarified. Much of the original research into nocturnal asthma has been performed or inspired by the participants at this meeting. We are most grateful to Napp Laboratories for sponsoring this first symposium on nocturnal asthma particularly to Dr Cyril Boroda, Medical Director and Janita Whittingham, Conference Co-ordinator, for all their help in arranging this meeting. We are also grateful to Dr Jonathan Levy for assisting in the preparation of this publication, which we hope will prove to be a useful 'state of the art' review of this complex topic.

References

Barnes, P.J. (1984). *Br. med. J.* 288, 1397.
Floyer, J. (1698). *A treatise of the asthma*. Wilkin, London.
Hetzel, M. (1981). *Thorax* **36**, 481.
Lancet (1983). Editorial. *Lancet* i, 220.
Turner-Warwick, M. (1977). *Br. J. resp. Dis.* **71**, 73.
Willis, T. (1679). *Pharmaceutice rationalis*, Vol. 2. Dring, Harper, Leigh, London.

The Definition and recognition of nocturnal asthma

M. TURNER-WARWICK

Brompton Hospital

In terms of the clinical history, the description 'episodic, wheezy, breathlessness' summarizes the most characteristic features of asthma. It is of some interest that Dodge and Burrows (1980) found that the question to patients which related most closely to that state in which they were observed objectively to have variable airflow limitation was 'do you have asthma?!' Thus most patients have little difficulty in recognizing asthma even if doctors contrive to make things difficult for themselves! Of course this does not deny the fact that important errors are made in individual patients and this occurs for a number of different reasons. A generally agreed definition useful for clinical purposes is 'a clinical syndrome characterized by partial airflow limitation which varies with time either spontaneously or as a result of treatment'. This definition is useful because it alerts doctors to the therapeutic opportunities. It is not designed to distinguish between those with and without associated conditions such as chronic bronchitis or emphysema. If, contrary to contemporary debate, the definition of asthma is relatively straightforward, the definition of 'nighttime' in the context of asthma (rather than the state of the moon!) is much more controversial. This is so for two reasons. First, it depends on what time you get up in the morning and, second, whether one wishes to distinguish between morning tightness and nocturnal attacks of asthma. There are many reasons for making such a distinction.

When considering nocturnal attacks of wheezy breathlessness, the major differential diagnosis is clearly between cardiac and bronchial asthma. Cardiac asthma does not usually present as a condition with recurrent morning 'dipping'. On the other hand it is characterized by orthopnoea and other evidence of left heart dysfunction. Nocturnal bronchial asthma forces the patient to sit up, but, between attacks, orthopnoea is not a feature unless there is in addition more persistent hyperinflation or continuing airflow limitation. Morning tightness on the other hand is very common.

Do nocturnal attacks and morning tightness occur in the same patients?

The standard questionnaire used for over 10 years in our asthma clinic includes the two questions 'do you get attacks of asthma at night?' and 'do you wake with a tight chest in the morning?'. Nocturnal asthma is very common, occurring overall in 75 per cent of a consecutive series of 395 new patients including children, adolescents, and adult asthmatics. This clinic population is probably representative of asthma clinics generally in this country because an exactly similar questionnaire was used concurrently by Dr Hugh Smyllie in Doncaster and, overall, 61 per cent of his patients reported nocturnal attacks. Nocturnal attacks are as common in children as in adults (Fig.1) but morning tightness tends to occur rather more frequently in older individuals (Fig.2).

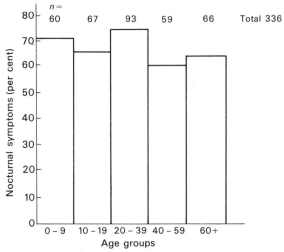

Fig. 1. *Age and nocturnal asthma.*

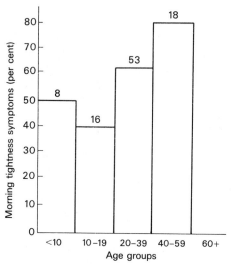

Fig. 2. *Age and morning tightness.*

Because house-dust mite hypersensitivity and nocturnal attacks of asthma are both common in childhood, it was tempting to suggest a cause-and-effect relationship. However in our overall experience nocturnal attacks were just as frequent in our skin-test-negative asthmatics as in our skin-test-positive ones (Table 1).

The distinction between nocturnal attacks and morning tightness may have other importance. The question of nocturnal asthma deaths will be considered by others in this volume and it may be important to differentiate between the risk factor of nocturnal asthma attacks (which must be acknowledged as extremely common) and the risk factor of morning dipping. We have analysed 100 patients to examine the

Table 1
Do you have asthma attacks at night?

	Nocturnal asthma present	Nocturnal asthma absent	Total
Skin test positive	238	78	316
(Row per cent)	75	25	
Skin test negative	56	23	79
(Row per cent)	71	29	
Total asthmatics	294	101	395
(Row per cent)	74	26	

relationship between nocturnal asthma and morning tightness. The results in Table 2 show that 27 per cent had nocturnal asthma only and 15 per cent morning tightness only.

If morning waking with severe asthma is different from nocturnal asthma, how does it develop? Contrary to obvious theoretical objections it has been possible to follow some patients through the night with peak flow recordings without destroying

Table 2
Nocturnal asthma and morning tightness

	Per cent ($n=99$)
Nocturnal asthma	71
Morning tightness	59
Both	44
Nocturnal asthma only	27
Morning tightness only	15
Neither	13

their pattern of morning dipping. In this study Dr Colin Soutar was able to demonstrate that the pattern throughout the night was variable. Some patients showed nocturnal variations as well as morning dipping but other individuals showed no nocturnal variability but striking morning dips. He also showed that there tended to be a gradual decline in the peak flow starting from about 1 a.m. but that this decline tended to become more precipitous at 5–6 a.m. He further showed it sometimes reversed spontaneously on or after waking in the morning. It was rapidly reversed by sympathomimetics and bronchodilators.

In conclusion, these are some of the features of asthma occurring during the hours of darkness and I hope that this will set the scene for the later chapters which will shed further light on the subject.

Reference

Dodge, R.R. and Burrows, B. (1980). The prevalence and incidence of asthma. Asthma like symptoms in a general population sample. *Am. Rev. resp. Dis.* **122**, 567.

Discussion

Professor C.M. Fletcher

I cannot accept that the history is adequate for the diagnosis of asthma. We cannot dispense with definitions altogether; the definition you gave is equally applicable to emphysema or severe reversible air flow obstruction but they do not respond markedly to treatment. There were some patients we label asthmatic who are resistant to steroids and to everything else, so we haven't yet got a definition that corresponds with what we say is asthma, but each time we use the word we should say in what sense we are using it.

Professor M. Turner-Warwick

I don't believe asthma by my definition is mutually exclusive with other disorders defined either in terms of anatomy, or symptoms of cough and sputum. I use the definition, as I think many other clinicians do, because it highlights a component of airways obstruction that is very important to identify with regard to management. If a patient with anatomical destructive emphysema has a variable component of his airways obstruction, there is no harm in labelling that patient as having emphysema (on the criteria that is used to define that condition) as well as asthma insofar as it highlights that they have something that you can treat. For research or clinical purposes, you can quantify that and specify a variation of 10, 15, 20 per cent, or whatever you like.

Professor D.C. Flenley

If we use words, let us at least use objective measurements and whoever reads the paper can decide what they want to call it.

Professor M. Turner-Warwick

There are a large number of cases which have been labelled emphysema, probably because the radiograph and full lung function suggest it, but this label may obscure the fact that they have a variable component as well.

Professor D.C. Flenley

You made a distinction between what the patient said they felt and what was measured with a peak flow meter. Did you imply that nocturnal asthma was what the patient told you in the morning they had?

Professor M. Turner-Warwick

> There is a conceptual definition which is variable air flow limitation. It may be measured by questionnaire form entirely or by waking the patient 2-hourly (or perhaps both).

Professor D.C. Flenley

> Could people have no nocturnal asthma on a questionnaire and yet have a 'morning dip'?

Professor M. Turner-Warwick

> I augmented the questionnaire with objective measurements, and have shown that this questionnaire has some validity.

Professor T.J. Clark

> I would like to support what Professor Turner-Warwick said about the heterogeneity of the mechanisms involved. I think there is little doubt both from formal studies and clinical experience that some patients respond to different drugs. There are patients who are steroid-resistant and others who appear to respond to steroids. Not only is there heterogeneity between patients but within patients; some patients may show a response to adding in a steroid, cromoglycate, or a different bronchodilator on one occasion and not on another. I think this heterogeneity will make any unitarian theory rather difficult to sustain.

Dr D.E. Stableforth

> In this clinical area where we seem to be preoccupied with, on the one hand, asthma with reversibility and on the other hand with emphysema and chronic bronchitis we should recognize that these conditions may occur together in the same patient. It is time we thought about a nomenclature for the disease which unifies the concept of airways obstruction which underlies all three conditions. You could then describe these as A (for airways obstruction), followed by R (for reversibility), E (for emphysema), S (for sputum), which could be graded. You would then give the clinician a real idea what you were talking about.

Professor B. Heard

> We studied the amount of airway smooth muscle in carefully selected asthmatics and bronchitics, and found that the volume of muscle in asthmatics was triple normal and in bronchitics double normal. These cases had been very carefully selected and there were one or two cases which we left out because they seemed to have asthma and chronic bronchitis. We used a detailed serial sections method to measure the muscle and we confirmed structurally that there was a hyperplasia of the muscle in chronic bronchitis. Some subsequent studies have failed to confirm this but they did not use serial sections.

Professor D.C. Flenley

You have not mentioned hyperreactivity.

Professor M. Turner-Warwick

With highly variable airway function, response to histamine may be difficult to interpret because of changes in the baseline. I have asked Freddie Hargreaves whether there is any advantage in doing a formal test of hyperreactivity when there is a period of peak flow showing high variability.

Dr N. McJohnson

Would you comment on the variability in peak flow rates at night in patients with left ventricular failure and paroxysmal nocturnal dyspnoea and how to differentiate that from asthma?

Professor M. Turner-Warwick

According to my definitions, there are two sorts of asthma — cardiac asthma and bronchial asthma — and they are both asthma because the airways are variable.

Asthma Deaths At Night

G.M. COCHRANE

New Cross and Guy's Hospitals, London, UK.

Introduction

For many centuries asthmatics have feared the nights. Dr John Floyer (1698) wrote 'I have observed the fit always to happen after sleep in the night when nerves are filled with windy Spirits and the heat of the bed has rarified the Spirits and Humours'! Before William Harvey's elucidation of the circulation most physicians considered paroxysmal nocturnal dyspnoea to be due to asthma and only after Harvey did physicians conjure the term 'cardiac asthma' for the frightening nocturnal breathlessness of pulmonary oedema. Asthma, despite being reported as the cause of death of over 1500 people per year in England and Wales since 1867, was considered a comparatively benign condition till the epidemic of deaths in the 1960s (Speizer *et al.* 1968). The rapid rise and fall in the asthma death rate, however, gave an awareness that even after the wane in epidemic deaths, there was a considerable mortality from asthma.

First report of asthma deaths at night in England and Wales

Cochrane and Clark (1975) analysed asthma deaths occurring in 1971 in the Greater London hospitals in the 35–64 year old age group, and determined that the majority of deaths were avoidable. These authors also observed that 13 deaths in hospital of the 19 attributable to asthma occurred between midnight and 8 a.m. In this study sedative drugs had been given to 15 of the patients and in four patients death followed in the ensuing 12 hours. A comparative control group of asthma 'survivors' also studied however, showed no significant difference in the frequency, amount, or type of sedative given. Sedation alone appeared not to be the primary cause of death at night but asthma was more likely to be mortally severe at night. The idea that asthma is more severe in the early hours of the morning was supported by the 'sudden death' of a patient with asthma, where peak flow measurements were recorded by the nurses (Fig. 1). Unfortunately, the data had been numerically recorded rather than graphically, and this 'sudden death' perhaps could have been anticipated and prevented.

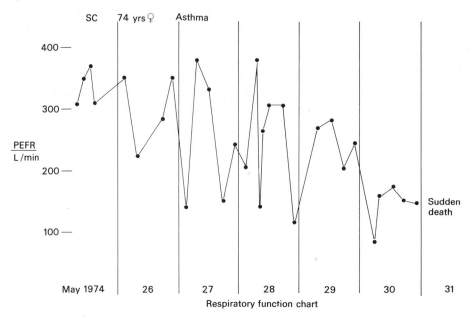

Fig. 1. *Peak flow recordings from a patient with asthma who died suddenly in the early hours of the morning. The data was originally only in numerical form in the nursing cardex.*

Do asthma deaths occur more commonly at night?

The initial study (Cochrane and Clark 1975) was followed by two excellent studies from Cardiff analysing asthma deaths in all age groups, both in and outside hospital. In the first (Macdonald *et al*. 1976*a*) 90 deaths due to asthma occurring outside hospitals were reported and it was suggested that the fatal attack was typically short but occurred in patients with a long history. Death was more common in those who had recently been discharged from hospital after a previous attack. The time of death was known in 79 of the 90 patients and showed no significant trend, but actual details of the time were not given nor was the method of analysis stated. The second paper (Macdonald *et al*. 1976 *b*) reported 53 deaths over the same period of time (1963–74) that occurred in hospital. The typical fatal attack had persisted for several days, but there was no obvious difference in severity of asthma between the patients in the two studies. The hour of death was known in 44 of the 53 subjects and again showed no significant trend. Twelve patients were given assisted ventilation and therefore the time of nocturnal death may have been obscured as no data is given of the time assisted ventilation was instituted.

Nocturnal bronchial hyperreactivity is dangerous!

Although the two Cardiff studies did not support the concept that nocturnal asthma was not only typical (Floyer 1698) but also dangerous, their conclusions were immediately contested. Hetzel *et al*, (1977) analysed sudden deaths and ventilatory arrests in hospital in-patients admitted with severe asthma. These authors noted that eight out of ten ventilatory arrests occurred between midnight and 8 a.m. This risk of sudden death or ventilatory arrest could not be correlated to the severity of the attack of asthma but it did correlate with the presence of marked diurnal variation in peak expiratory flow rate (PEFR). Patients who were noted to have excessive falls in the early morning PEFR or who woke in the early hours of the morning with breathlessness or wheeze were at risk of sudden death. Two deaths after a sudden attack of asthma in young people were reported by Bateman and Clarke (1979) from a clinic set up to identify and manage such 'at risk' patients. Both these patients had been shown to have marked diurnal variation in PEFR and were considered to have excessive bronchial hyperreactivity. These authors concluded 'a wide diurnal variation in PEFR may well be a better guide to recognition of the susceptible patient than the factors previously mentioned' (length of history, age of onset, allergic factors, etc.).

Bronchial hyperreactivity is dangerous but does it lead to asthma deaths at night?

Fifty-three more asthma deaths in Birmingham (Ormerod and Stableforth 1980) occurring both in and out of hospital, again reflected the abysmal treatment of asthmatics and echoed the original observations (Speizer *et al.* 1968; Cochrane and Clark 1975; Macdonald *et al.* 1976 *a, b*) that many deaths were avoidable. Ormerod and Stableforth (1980) highlighted the inadequacy of death certification, a point noted by Cochrane and Clark (1975) but also observed that 'the previously reported trend of deaths in hospital occurring in the early hours is not shown by this survey'.

Published data in *The Lancet* (1983) analyses four studies (Cochrane and Clark 1975; Macdonald *et al.* 1976 *a, b*; British Thoracic Association 1982) and reported that 93 of 219 asthmatic deaths occurred between midnight and 8 a.m. Deaths from any cause are more likely at night but are in excess by only 5 per cent of the rest of the day, but deaths recorded from asthma are 28 per cent more likely to occur at night.

The British Thoracic Association (1982) prospectively organised a study of death from asthma in two regions of England. This superb study showed that 80 of the 90 deaths were associated with avoidable factors. However, their original report did not reveal the time of death but this is due to be published shortly. Provisional data (personal communication) suggests that nearly two-thirds of the deaths occurred between 8 p.m. and 8 a.m. — a level far in excess of that anticipated. If one also considers ventilator deaths which have frequently occurred before official death is considered to have taken place, death from asthma would appear to be more frequent at night.

Causes of nocturnal deaths from asthma

Nearly ten years ago, Cochrane and Clark (1975) observed an increase in nocturnal deaths from asthma and sedative drugs appeared to be implicated. Respiratory depressant therapy can no longer be considered a factor as more recent studies have shown. Bronchial hyperreactivity and diurnal variation in asthma appear more likely factors. All the studies have suggested poor assessment of the severity of an attack of asthma by patient and clinician. Although patients are frequently considered to be poorly aware of the severity of their asthma, up to 80 per cent are more efficient in assessing their asthma than the physician. A way of determining the appreciation of severity of asthma by a patient is to examine his request for medical advice. The majority of chest clinics have a direct referral advice system but do patients seek advice through this system and are their symptoms worse at night? Horn and Cochrane (unpubished data) investigated the time of day at which patients with various symptoms seek advice from an accident and emergency department in London. Many factors determine the time a patient seeks advice: even the prospect of not waiting for hours may lead a patient to choose a 3 a.m. appointment rather than an official family practitioner appointment at 9 a.m. Analysis of patients presenting to an accident and emergency department shows that a marked preponderance of patients who present at night do so with severe breathlessness. The pattern of presentation to a casualty department is shown in Fig. 2. The majority of

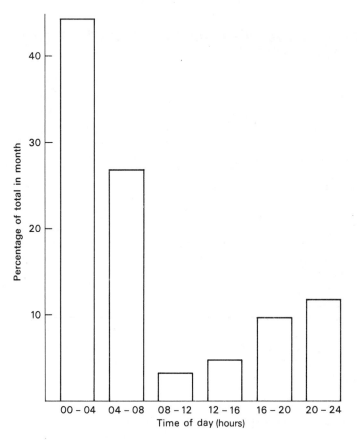

Fig. 2. Presentation to Guy's casualty during November 1983 with acute respiratory symptoms. The number of patients presenting in four-weekly periods during the day has been corrected for the total number presenting during the same period, and then expressed as a percentage of the total.

these patients had severe airflow obstruction compatible with a diagnosis of asthma. Comparative data with other diseases, such as abdominal pain, suggest that, even if asthma death is not more common at night, attacks of asthma requiring urgent advice from an accident and emergency department are.

Conclusion

Asthma deaths still occur and appear to be avoidable in 80–85 per cent of the reported incidents. There appears to be a higher incidence of death at night, although some authors may still dispute this. Diurnal variation of asthma with more severe symptoms at night and coincidental fall in PEFR suggests that in the 'brittle' asthmatic nighttime may be more dangerous. Therapy aimed at reducing diurnal hyperreactivity (Horn *et al*. 1984) may diminish the unacceptably high incidence of death from asthma.

References

Bateman, J.R. and Clarke, S.W. (1979). *Thorax*34, 40.
British Thoracic Association (1982). *Br. med. J.* **285**, 1251.
Cochrane, G.M. and Clarke, T.J.H. (1975). *Thorax* **30**, 300.
Floyer, J. (1698). *A treatise of the asthma*. Wilkin, London.
Hetzel, M.R., Clark, T.J.H. and Branthwaite, M.A. (1977). *Br. med. J.* **i**, 808.
Horn, C.R., Clark, T.J.H., and Cochrane, G.M. (1984). *Thorax*(in press).
Lancet(1983). Editorial. *Lancet* **i**, 220–2.
Macdonald, J.B., Seaton, A. and Williams, D.A. (1976 *a*). *Br. med. J.* **i**, 1493.
Macdonald, J.B., Macdonald, E.T., Seaton, A., and Williams, D.A. (1976 *b*). *Br. med. J.* **ii**, 721.
Omerod, L.P. and Stableforth D.E. (1980). *Br. med. J.* **i**, 687.
Speizer, F.E., Doll, R., and Heaf, P. (1968). *Br. med. J.* **i**, 335.

Discussion

Dr M. Hetzel

I do not think we should be too concerned about the actual time of death in these people and we want to be looking for a relationship between severe nocturnal asthma and sudden death. These patients who have very severe nocturnal asthma are in a very precarious and labile position and it is not unreasonable to expect that they might die relatively suddenly at any time of day. We should not be too worried therefore if we are not necessarily seeing a very strong association with increased sudden death at night.

Dr G.M. Cochrane

I agree that if they have a high degree of bronchial lability patients are obviously more at risk, but it would appear they are even more likely to die at night when their peak flow is low. In our latest survey, nearly 10 years after the first survey, there were no deaths in which sedatives were implicated.

Professor M. Turner-Warwick

You said that in the BTA study 80 of the 93 deaths were avoidable and that many might be related to 'morning dips'. Does this imply that because the patient had a 'morning dip' asthma is avoidable?

Dr G.M. Cochrane

'Morning dips' do appear to increase the risk of death if you take the little data that is available with peak flow measurements such as the data of Bateman and Clark and the 'one off' cases that I think we have all got.

Professor M. Turner-Warwick

There are a lot of patients with severe 'morning dipping' that all your drugs cannot control.

Dr G.M. Cochrane

Some patients will have a drop in peak flow but others will wake up with severe nocturnal symptoms without much drop; we have one patient who has a peak flow drop of less than 40 out of 400 overnight, with severe nocturnal symptoms and the only way we showed that this was 'asthma' was by making measurements of

his chest when he woke and he had increased his chest measurement by 2 inches.

Dr D.E. Stableforth

I think that you put too strong an interpretation on the conclusions of the BTA study with regard to avoidability of death from
asthma. What it said was that avoidable factors were present in
the deaths of 80 per cent of patients which if different might not
have resulted in the death of a patient ultimately, which is not the
same as saying that 80 per cent of the deaths were avoidable.

Dr G.M. Cochrane

From our own study we felt that 85 per cent of deaths were
avoidable.

Dr N. Wilson

I am still a little confused about 'morning dip' and how it differs
from nocturnal asthma. Is it right to say that the dangerous type
of 'morning dipping' is when the inhalers no longer work during
the night or they have to be used several times? Would that be
more useful as a concept, because the patient without a peak flow
meter can then be told that when their nocturnal symptoms do
not reverse easily they should seek help? That would differentiate between the 'morning dips' which are apparently steroid-
resistant and commonly seen.

Dr G.M. Cochrane

I agree and I think you have to use symptoms, waking at night,
frequency of bronchodilator use, and, if applicable, peak flow.

Dr I.S. Petheram

One factor not mentioned is accessibility of patients to medical
care when they are in trouble. Two patients I am most worried
about at the moment are two young women who have been into
hospital with sudden catastrophic asthma which recovered with
the usual treatment. They live over 20 miles from the Casualty
Department and they have a 'morning dipping' pattern which is
refractory to all the drugs I have tried so far. The only practical
advice I have given them is to try moving to town.

Dr G.M. Cochrane

Both Stuart Clark and I have published data on patients who are
very severe and cannot get help rapidly. We advise subcutaneous, self-administered injections. We have two patients
who have managed to survive on that and get to hospital.

Dr C.K. Connolly

I was a member of the research committee of the BTA study. I think that it is important to re-emphasise that all that was said was that there were apparently avoidable factors in the majority of deaths. The assumption that good control will in fact reduce death rate worries me and the death rate has not been reduced over the last 10 years, despite the fact that control of the majority of moderately severe asthmatics has improved over this time. Are we absolutely certain that control of symptoms will in fact reduce the death rate?

Dr G.M. Cochrane

No, but we haven't actually achieved that state so I don't think I can answer the question. Asthma is grossly underdiagnosed and in some surveys these patients have died without receiving drugs. Furthermore some patients who are known to have asthma are not treated in a way which most of us would think is the minimum.

Interactions of asthma and sleep

N.J. DOUGLAS

University of Edinburgh and Edinburgh Royal Infirmary, Edinburgh, UK.

Many asthmatics report that they are awoken from sleep by cough or wheeze, yet there have been surprisingly few studies of whether sleep causes nocturnal asthma. This chapter deals with possible direct interactions of sleep and asthma; indirect association such as sleep contributing to the control of circadian variation in hormone levels or bronchial reactivity will be covered elsewhere.

Does sleep cause nocturnal asthma?

There have as yet been no measurements of airway calibre in sleeping patients with nocturnal asthma. Several groups have studied forced expiratory flow rates in such patients but, as these clearly cannot be measured in sleeping patients, these studies have limited relevance to the effect of sleep on nocturnal asthma.

However, such studies (Turner-Warwick 1977; Clark and Hetzel 1977; Hetzel and Clark 1979) confirm a fact that is obvious clinically, namely that nocturnal bronchospasm persists after the patient awakes. This almost certainly means that a direct sleep-related neurological reflex is not the sole cause of nocturnal asthma as functions which are so controlled — e.g. the breathing pattern (Douglas *et al*, 1982 *a*) and ventilatory control (Douglas *et al*, 1982 *b*, *c*) — return to the levels found in wakefulness coincidental with arousal.

Forced expiratory flow rates could also determine whether sleep is essential for the production of nocturnal asthma. Hetzel and Clark (1979) kept 11 asthmatics with documented morning dips awake until 3, 4, or 5 a.m. and then allowed them to sleep until 6 a.m.

They compared the peak flow rate decrease from 10 p.m. until 3, 4 or 5 a.m. with the subsequent decrease while the patient slept (Fig. 1). In six patients almost all the decrease in flow rate occurred prior to sleep, whereas in the remaining five the reverse happened and most of the decrease in flow rate occurred during the one to three hours when sleep was permitted. This study is further complicated by the fact that during the 'awake' period, the subjects 'went to bed at 22.00 and adopted the sleeping posture ... reading or listening to the radio'. It would be extremely difficult for most subjects to totally avoid brief naps or 'microsleeps' in such a situation, and it is not clear how rigorously the patients were observed during this period. The most that can be concluded from this study is that sleep may be important in the pathogenesis of nocturnal bronchoconstriction in some patients, and that very short periods of sleep might be sufficient to produce these effects.

The same workers (Clark and Hetzel 1977) showed that the change from day to

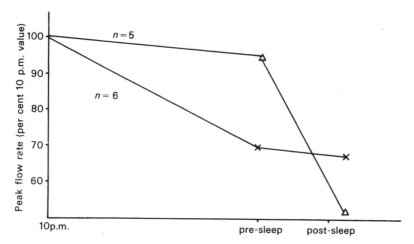

Fig. 1. *Change in peak flow between 10 p.m. and sleep onset (at 3, 4, or 5 a.m.) and the subsequent change during sleep in 11 morning dippers. (Plotted from the data in Hetzel and Clark (1979).)*

night shift is rapidly accompanied by inversion of the circadian rhythm in peak flow, and that this 'was complete by the time the first natural sleep had taken place as each new shift started'. Thus, the circadian rhythm of flow rate is synchronous with the sleep–wake cycle, but this does not prove that sleep causes nocturnal asthma.

Is nocturnal asthma related to specific stages of sleep?

Several groups have recorded the electroencephalogram during sleep in such patients and noted from which sleep stage patients were awakened with attacks of asthma. One early study (Ravenscroft and Hartmann 1968) found that the patients were awakened more frequently from REM sleep than would be expected by chance. However, this study was only published in abstract and has not been confirmed by subsequent observations (Kales *et al.* 1968, 1970; Montplaisir *et al.* 1982). In by far the largest of these studies, including 93 'asthmatic episodes', Kales *et al.* (1968) found that asthmatic attacks were randomly distributed throughout the stages of sleep in proportion to the amount of time spent in each sleep stage(Fig.2). Studies suggesting that deep sleep (stages 3 and 4 sleep) may protect against asthma attacks are based on too little data to allow this conclusion to be made (Kales *et al.* 1970; Monplaisir *et al.* 1982). All of these studies must be interpreted with caution as the 'asthmatic episodes' were usually loosely defined and the effect of sleep stage on arousal thresholds is poorly understood.

Interest in the possible effect of sleep stage on bronchomotor tone has been further stimulated by the observation that in tracheostomized dogs, bronchial calibre becomes markedly variable during REM sleep (Sullivan *et al.* 1979). This variability was, however, random with no consistent tendency either to bronchoconstriction or bronchodilation. Lopes *et al.* (1983) reported that, in normal man, pulmonary resistance is increased in non-REM sleep, returning in REM sleep to levels similar to those in wakefulness. However, changes in pulmonary resistance may reflect upper airway flaccidity during sleep rather than changes in bronchomotor tone. Further, this data is based on measurements made using an induction stethogram; this device has not been validated for accurate measurements of respired volumes during sleep and its ability to record expiratory flow rates — which are critical to the measurement of pulmonary resistance — is under question even in immobile awake subjects

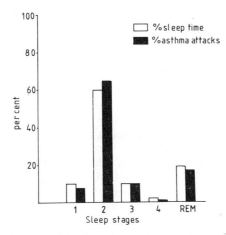

Fig. 2. Percentage of (a) sleep spent in various sleep stages (open rectangles) and (b) percentage of asthmatic attacks arousing the patient from each sleep stage (shaded rectangles). (Data plotted from Kales et al. (1968).)

(Mannix *et al*. 1984). As yet, there have been no measurements of bronchomotor tone in different sleep stages in sleeping asthmatics, the nearest being a study in which eight asthmatics were deliberately awoken from either REM or non-REM sleep during two nights in a sleep laboratory, and asked to perform a forced expiratory manoeuvre immediately on waking (Shapiro *et al*. 1982). Analysis of the FEV_1s obtained from time-matched wakenings in each subject showed that FEV_1 was lower when patients were awoken from REM than from non-REM sleep. However, this difference was only 200 ml compared to an overnight fall in FEV_1 of around 800 ml and it appears that time-related factors are far more important than any sleep-stage-dependent differences.

It must be remembered that the conclusion of this study that airways are narrower in REM than non-REM sleep is contrary to the evidence in normal man (Lopes *et al*. 1983). Thus further measurements of airflow resistance in both normal subjects and asthmatics during sleep are required to clarify this unlikely discrepancy.

Studies of breathing and oxygenation during sleep

Several groups have recently studied oxygenation and breathing patterns in sleeping asthmatics. Stable asthmatics with nocturnal wheeze exhibit mild hypoxaemia during sleep (Montplaisir *et al*. 1982; Tabachnik *et al*. 1981; Catterall *et al*. 1982, 1983; Morgan *et al*. 1983), but arterial oxygen saturation rarely falls below 85 per cent. Although the changes in arterial oxygen saturation during sleep — from awake saturation to the lowest level recorded during sleep — are greater in asthmatics than in age- and sex-matched controls (Montplaisir *et al.* 1982; Catterall *et al.* 1982), calculated changes in arterial oxygen tension are similar in asthmatics and normal subjects at about 2.7 kPa, the greater desaturation in asthmatics reflecting their lower starting point on the oxygen haemoglobin dissociation curve. Thus stable asthmatics do not exhibit excessive nocturnal hypoxaemia such as might occur if they had marked bronchospasm during sleep.

It is unclear whether asthmatics breathe more irregularly during sleep than age-, sex- and weight-matched normal subjects. We found a small but significant increase in such irregular breathing in asthmatics, due almost entirely to the asthmatics having more apnoeas (Catterall *et al.* 1982), but Montplaisir and colleagues (1982) found no such difference. The increase in apnoeas in our own study may have been because it was performed in the summer and many of the patients may have had mild rhinitis, nasal obstruction now being known to increase apnoeas (Zwillich *et al.* 1981; McNicholas *et al.* 1982). Further, our asthmatics had impaired sleep quality with more arousals and an increased amount of drowsiness and this would also predispose to apnoeas. These apnoeas were, however, brief and were not associated with undue hypoxia and thus their clinical significance is doubtful.

The changes in mean ventilation from wakefulness to the different sleep stages are similar in asthmatics (Catterall *et al.* 1983; Morgan *et al.* 1983) and normal subjects, (Douglas *et al.* 1982*a*), the lowest level of ventilation occurring in REM sleep, then averaging around 80 per cent of the ventilation in wakefulness. Expiratory time, which might be prolonged during bronchospasm, was initially thought to be prolonged during REM sleep (Catterall *et al.* 1982). However, subsequent measurements in a larger number of patients (Morgan *et al.* 1983) have shown that although expiratory time is more variable in REM sleep, there is no overall change in mean expiratory time in any sleep stage in asthmatics (Fig. 3).

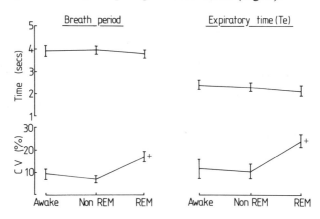

Fig. 3. Breath period and expiratory time (upper panels) and their respective variability indicated as coefficient of variation. + = P<0.01.

Thus although studies on sleeping asthmatics have not included any measurements of airway calibre, the indirect evidence, such as the lack of excess hypoxia, similar changes in ventilation in asthmatics compared to normal subjects, and the fact that expiratory time does not change between sleep stages in asthmatics, does not suggest that marked bronchoconstriction occurs during specific sleep stages in such patients. However, there is an obvious need for more direct measurements of airway calibre in sleeping asthmatics.

The effect of sleep on protective responses to an asthmatic attack

If, for whatever reason, a patient has an attack of nocturnal asthma when asleep, the normal ventilatory protective responses will be impaired. The patient will be hypoxic and hypoventilating because he is asleep and both the hypoxic (Douglas *et al.* 1982*b*; Berthon-Jones and Sullivan 1982; Hedemark and Kronenberg 1982) and hypercapnic (Douglas *et al.* 1982 *c*; Hedemark and Kronenberg 1982) ventilatory responses will be reduced, the maximal fall being to about one-third of the waking levels in REM sleep. The effect of sleep on the ventilatory responses to added respiratory loads has not been studied in detail, but there is some evidence (Iber *et al.* 1982) that this is impaired in non-REM sleep, no measurements having been made in REM sleep.

These factors may well allow patients who have attacks of nocturnal asthma to develop significant hypoxia and hypercapnia if these attacks occur during sleep and probably such attacks are only prevented from being fatal by the patient's arousal. There have been no studies of the causes of arousal in attacks of nocturnal asthma. In normal subjects it is known that both hypoxia (Douglas *et al.* 1982 *b*; Berthon-Jones and Sullivan 1982; Hedemark and Kronenberg 1982; Gothe *et al.* 1982) and hypercapnia (Douglas *et al.* 1982*c*; Hedemark and Kronenberg 1982) are relatively poor stimuli to arousal. Similarly, neither the addition of an inspiratory resistance (Iber *et al.* 1982) nor total occlusion of inspiration (Issa and Sullivan 1983) result in rapid arousal from non-REM sleep. The arousal from REM with airway occlusion is far more rapid (6.2 ± 2.7 (SD) sec) than from non-REM sleep (20.4 ± 7.6 sec; $P<0.001$) when many subjects do not arouse until more than 30 seconds after total occlusion of their airway. Thus, when asthmatic attacks start when the patient is asleep, impaired ventilatory responses and poor arousal responses may mean that the attack can progress further prior to the patient initiating treatment or seeking assistance than when similar attacks occur with the patient awake.

The effect of asthma on sleep

As any patient with nocturnal asthma will verify, asthmatics do not sleep as well as normal subjects. This has been documented by EEG recording (Kales *et al.* 1968; Montplaisir *et al.* 1982; Catterall *et al.* 1982) the major difference being that asthmatics have an increased amount of intervening wakefulness and drowsiness. In one of these studies (Kales *et al.* 1968) the patients were receiving oral ephedrine and theophyllines which may have interfered with sleep (Rhind *et al.* 1984) but in the other two studies, no such oral medications were being received and so the impaired sleep quality presumably reflects their asthma.

Effects of sleep deprivation on ventilatory responses

Many asthmatics have slept poorly or not at all on the nights preceding admission to hospital with acute severe asthma. It has recently been found (Cooper and Phillips 1982; White *et al.* 1983; Schiffman *et al.* 1983) that such sleep deprivation decreases the ventilatory responses to both hypoxia and hypercapnia by about 25 per cent, although the ventilatory response to an inspiratory resistance seems to be unaffected by sleep deprivation (Schiffman *et al.* 1983). These decreases in ventilatory responses may, along with exhaustion, help to explain why patients with acute severe asthma sometimes develop hypoventilation.

Conclusions

1. It is not known whether sleep causes nocturnal asthma.
2. Ventilation and protective ventilatory responses are reduced during sleep and this may increase the risks in nocturnal asthma.
3. Asthma disrupts sleep.

References

Berthon-Jones, M. and Sullivan, C.E. (1982). *Am. Rev. resp. Dis.* **125**, 632.
Catterall, J.R., Douglas, N.J., Calverley, P.M.A., *et al.* (1982). *Lancet* **i**, 301.
—— Morgan, A.D., Douglas, N.J., *et al.* (1983). *Am. Rev. resp. Dis.* **127**, Suppl. 106.
Clark, T.J.H., and Hetzel, M.R. (1977). *Br. J. Dis. Chest* **71**, 87.
Cooper, K.R., and Phillips, B.A. (1982). *J. Appl. Physiol.* **53**, 855.
Douglas, N.J., White, D.P., Pickett, C.K., Weil, J.V., and Zwillich, C.W. (1982 *a*). *Thorax* **37**, 840.
——, ——, Weil, J.V., *et al.* (1982 *b*). *Am. Rev. resp. Dis.* **125**, 286.
——, ——, ——, Pickett, C.K., and Zwillich, C.W.(1982 *c*). *Am. Rev. resp. Dis.* **126**, 758.
Gothe, B., Goldman, M.D., Cherniak, N.S., and Mantey, P. (1982). *Am. Rev. resp. Dis.* **126**, 97.
Hedemark, L.L., and Kronenberg, R.S. (1982). *J. Appl. Physiol.* **53**, 307.
Hetzel, M.R., and Clark, T.J.H. (1979). *Thorax* **34**, 749.
Iber, C., Berssenbrugge, A., Skatrud, J.B., and Dempsey, J.A. (1982). *J. Appl. Physiol.* **52**, 607.
Issa, F.G., and Sullivan, C.E. (1983). *J. Appl. Physiol.* **55**, 1113.
Kales, A., Beall, G.N., Bajor, G.F., Jacobson, A., and Kales, J.D. (1968). *J. Allerg.* **41**, 164.
——, Kales, J.D., Sly, R.M., Scharf, M.B., Tan, T. and Preston, T.A. (1970). *J. Allerg.* **46**, 300.
Lopes, J.M., Tabachnik, E., Muller, N.L., Levison, H., and Bryan, A.C. (1983). *J. Appl. Physiol.* **54**, 773.
Mannix, S.E., Chowienczyk, P., Barnes, P.J., and Pride, N.B. (1984). *Clin. Sci.* **66**, 58P.
McNicholas, W.T., Tarlo, S., Cole, P., *et al.* (1982). *Am. Rev. resp. Dis.* **126**, 625.
Montplaisir, J., Walsh, J., and Malo, J.L. (1982). Nocturnal asthma: features of attacks, sleep and breathing patterns.*Am. Rev. resp. Dis.* **125**, 18–22.
Morgan, A.D., Connaughton, J.J., Catterall, J.R., Shapiro, C.M., Douglas, N.J., and Flenley, D.C. (1983). Effects of sodium cromoglycate on nocturnal asthma. *Clin Sci.* **65**, 7P.
Ravenscroft, K., and Hartmann, E.L. (1968). The temporal correlation of nocturnal asthmatic attacks and the D-state. *Psychophysiology* **4**, 396–7.
Rhind, G.B., Connaughton, J.J., McFie, J., Douglas, N.J., and Flenley, D.C., (1984). The effects of theophylline on nocturnal wheeze and sleep quality in adults with asthma. *Am. Rev. resp. Dis.* (abstract in press).
Schiffman, P.L., Trontel, M.C., Mazar, M.F., and Edelman, N.H. (1983). Sleep deprivation decreases ventilatory response to CO_2 but not load compensation. *Chest* **84**, 695–8.
Shapiro, C.M., Montgomery, I., and Catterall, J.R. (1982). Breathing, bronchoconstriction and sleep in nocturnal asthma. *Thorax* **37**, 238–9.
Sullivan, C.E., Zamel, N., Kozar, L.F., Murphy, E., and Phillipson, E.A. (1979). Regulation of airway smooth muscle tone in sleeping dogs. *Am. Rev. resp. Dis.* **119**, 87–98.
Tabachnik, E., Muller, N.L., Levison, H., and Bryan, A.C. (1981). Chest wall mechanics and pattern of breathing during sleep in asthmatic adolescents. *Am. Rev. resp. Dis.* **124**, 269–3.
Turner-Warwick, M. (1977). On observing patterns of airflow obstruction in chronic asthma. *Br. J. Dis. Chest* **71**, 73–76.
White, D.P., Douglas, N.J., Pickett, C.K., Zwillich, C.W., and Weil, J.V. (1983). Sleep deprivation and the control of ventilation. *Am. Rev. resp. Dis.* **128**, 984–6.
Zwillich, C.W., Pickett, C., Hanson, F.N., and Weil, J.V. (1981). Disturbed sleep and prolonged apnoea during nasal obstruction in normal men. *Am. Rev. resp. Dis.* **124**, 158–60.

Discussion

Professor M. Turner-Warwick

From the clinical point of view did the asthmatics you studied complain of nocturnal asthma?

Dr N.J. Douglas

They were all patients who said that they had nocturnal asthma, and were studied on a run-in period of two weeks and shown to have 'morning dipping' as defined before and after peak flow rates. They all reported that they woke up through the night with asthmatic attacks.

Professor M. Turner-Warwick

You suggested that asthma attacks might disturb the sleep but it might be the sympathomimetics and other drugs that were being taken that disturbed the sleep rather than the disease.

Dr N.J. Douglas

I agree and we have further data that supports that drugs do disturb sleep, but the study is not yet complete.

Professor T.J. Clark

Previous work suggests that deep sleep is not very commonly associated with asthmatic attacks and there are many patients who are treated with sedatives. Have you got any observations on the role of sedatives, such as ketotifen, in either generating asthmatic attacks or appropriately stopping them?

Dr N. J. Douglas

The data of Kales in children and Montplaisir in adults drew conclusions that I think are invalid because of insufficient data. Deep sleep, as defined by stage 3 and 4, only occurs during 15 per cent of the night and they were dealing with a very low number of asthmatic awakenings. Kales's study in adults has a far larger number of awakenings and showed that deep sleep is as bad as any other stage. Ketotifen didn't seem to do anything particularly bad to the asthma and they slept marginally better, but it is certainly not a panacea for nocturnal asthma.

Dr P.J. Barnes

We really do need to know what happens to airway tone at night without waking people up. As you pointed out, using the differentiated respitrace signal to measure air flow is a very inadequate means of doing this, so we have been trying to develop a more direct method of measuring air flow during the night. Until we have the information of the natural history of airway tone at night in both normal and asthmatics it is rather difficult to interpret the results of waking people up suddenly, particularly when you consider that arousal is probably a very important factor. You may be quite bronchoconstricted but with a low arousal and so you wouldn't wake up and it wouldn't be recognized that you were bronchoconstricted at that time. Both arousal and bronchoconstriction need to be sorted out and the only way that can be done is by making nondisturbing measurements of airway tone at night.

Professor D.C. Flenley

I agree, but the problem is the method. Unlike patients with the sleep apnoea syndrome, asthmatics will not tolerate moderately invasive procedures well. Of course, if you do something that stops the character sleeping you have lost the very thing you are studying.

Dr G.M. Sterling

Do we know the effect of hypoxia on bronchomotor tone in asthmatics?

Professor D.C. Flenley

Hypercapnia causes bronchoconstriction but it is nothing like the level that occurs in the asthmatics.

Dr G.M. Sterling

But it may not be the hypercapnia so much as the hyperventilation. There is a much stronger stimulus in the asthmatic or a much greater effect in the asthmatic than in the normal.

Mucociliary clearance at night — effect of physical activity, posture, and circadian rhythm

D. PAVIA

Department of Thoracic Medicine, The Royal Free Hospital and School of Medicine, London NW3 2QG, UK.

Introduction

The removal of inhaled particulate matter and intrinsic biological debris from the tracheobronchial tree is achieved by the mucociliary escalator with cough acting as a reserve.

Mucociliary clearance is a primary lung defence mechanism which may be modified by temperature (Guillerm *et al.* 1966), humidity (Hirsch *et al.* 1975), physical exercise (Wolff *et al.* 1977), cigarette smoking (Lourenço *et al.* 1971), and pharmacological agents (Pavia *et al.* 1983). Its effectiveness has been reported to decrease with age (Goodman *et al.* 1978; Puchelle *et al.* 1979) and is depressed in patients with asthma (Bateman *et al.* 1983) and chronic bronchitis (Pavia *et al.* 1983). Little is known, however, of its physiological control.

Asthmatic patients often demonstrate a nocturnal deterioration of their airflow obstruction (Clark and Hetzel 1977) as well as irregular breathing patterns at night with accompanying falls of their oxygen saturation unrelated to sleep apnoea (Catterall *et al.* 1982). Furthermore, some studies have reported an increased incidence of non-fatal respiratory arrests and deaths at night (Cochrane and Clark 1975; Hetzel *et al.* 1977).

Studies are reviewed here of the effects of physical activity, posture, circadian rhythm, anad sleep on the clearance of tracheobronchial secretions in healthy human subjects and in patients with mild but stable asthma previously reported elsewhere (Bateman *et al.* 1978 *a, b*).

Subjects and patients

In the studies on healthy subjects there were 10 volunteers (five male, five female; six non-smokers, and four current cigarette smokers) with normal lung function. Their physical characteristics, cigarette consumption, and ventilatory function are summarized in Table 1.

In the studies on asthmatics there were 10 patients (eight male, two female) with mild but stable asthma (who all had documented nocturnal symptoms from previous hospital admissions). Seven of the patients were non-smokers, two were current smokers, and one was an ex-cigarette smoker. Their maintenance medication was inhaled bronchodilators which were omitted for at least 12 hours prior to, and

Table 1

Mean ± SE physical characteristics, tobacoo consumption, and ventilatory function for two groups: 10 healthy subjects and 10 mild but stable asthmatics

	Healthy Subjects	Asthma Patients
Age (years)	30±7	34±4
Height (m)	1.67±0.05	1.71±0.03
weight (kg)	62±9	70±4
Cigarette consumtion (pk-yr)	2±4	39±25
predicted FEV (per cent)*	121±8	71±7
predicted FVC (per cent) *	118±8	88±5
predicted PEFR (per cent) *	101±7	70±7
predicted MMFR (25–75 (per cent)*	—	49±8
predicted $\dot{V}_{max}$ 25 (per cent)†	—	26±4
predicted $\dot{V}_{max}$ 50 (per cent)†	—	35±6

*Batemann *et al*. 1978 *a*. †Cotes (1975).

during, the six-hour tracheobronchial clearance observation periods. Their physical characteristics, cigarette consumption and ventilatory function are also shown in Table 1; they had a moderate degree of large-airways obstruction with considerably impaired small-airways function.

Informed, written consent was obtained from all subjects prior to the commencement of the studies.

Methods

Tracheobronchial mucociliary clearance

Tracheobronchial mucociliary clearance was measured by an objective, non-invasive radioaerosol tracer method which has been described elsewhere (Pavia *et al*. 1980). Polystyrene microspheres of 5μ diameter, firmly tagged (Few *et al*. 1970) with the gamma-emitting radionuclide $^{99}Tc^m$ ($t_{1/2}=6$ h), were inhaled via the mouth (whilst wearing a nose clip) under strictly controlled conditions. The initial deposition and subsequent retention of the deposited radioaerosol in both lungs was monitored by scintillation detector(s) suitably positioned over the chest (Thomson *et al*. 1973).

The detector(s) was placed within a wide-angle lead collimator so that the field of view included most of both lungs but excluded the stomach. In the daytime active runs counting was performed by two opposing scintillation detectors located anteriorly and posteriorly to the chest at the level of the midpoint of the sternum with each subject seated. A count was made immediately after inhalation and thereafter at half-hourly intervals for a total of six hours, with a final count at 24 hours post-inhalation. The proportion of the radioaerosol retained at 24 hours was taken to represent that proportion of the lung burden which had been deposited beyond the reach of the cilia (i.e. alveolar deposition) and was therefore not available for mucus clearance (Cammer and Philipson 1978). Counts at the same time intervals were also collected in the two supine awake studies. However, on these occasions only one scintillation detector was used which was placed anteriorly and centrally over the chest of the supine healthy subjects. In the sleep studies counts were taken in the erect posture immediately after inhalation and at 0.5, 6, and 24 hours thereafter. The radioactivity counts were corrected for background and radioactive decay and expressed as a percentage of the inital count in any one study in order to adjust for unavoidable differences in the initial lung burden. The initial lung burden did not exceed 30 μCi in any one run; this was estimated to result in an absorbed lung dose of the order of 12 mrem.

The initial topographical distribution of the radioaerosol within the lungs was obtained immediately following inhalation using a rectilinear gamma scanner (Dawson *et al*. 1971). The topographical distribution was expressed quantitatively in terms of a penetration index (PI) which was arbitrarily defined as the amount of radioactivity present in the outer 2/5 of the right lung divided by that present in the inner 2/5.

Ventilatory function

In the case of the healthy subjects, the forced vital capacity (FVC), the forced expiratory volume in 1 s (FEV_1), and the peak expiratory flow rate (PEFR) were measured 1 hour prior to each study.

For the asthmatic patients measurements were additionally made of maximum mid-expiratory flow rate (MMFR $_{25-75}$) and flow rates at 25 and 50 per cent of VC ($\dot{V}_{max}25$, $\dot{V}_{max}50$) — again approximately 1 hour prior to each study. PEFR was measured using a Wright peak expiratory flow meter. FVC, FEV_1, and MMFR $_{25-75}$ were measured using a dry bellows spirometer (Vitalograph). $\dot{V}_{max}25$ and $\dot{V}_{max}50$ were measured from maximal flow-volume (air) curves using a waterless, piston/cylinder-type spirometer (Ohio 840) and a Bryans X–Y plotter.

Statistical analysis

The data of the variables measured in these studies were not normally distributed, so the Wilcoxon test for pair differences was used in the statistical analyses.

Study design

Each healthy subject completed four studies in a random order and separated by several days: (1) daytime awake with normal physical activity, eating, and drinking (daytime active); (2) daytime awake, supine and fasting (daytime supine); (3) nighttime awake, supine and fasting (nighttime awake); and (4) nighttime asleep.

Each asthmatic patient completed two studies in a random order and separated by one to three weeks (1) daytime active; (2) nighttime asleep.

All studies commenced approximately at midday or midnight. In the supine studies the subjects, under continuous observation, remained supine for approximately 5.5 h from 0.5 to 6.0 hours post-radioaerosol inhalation. They took neither food nor drink for one hour before inhaling the radioaerosol and for the following six hours. The three supine studies were conducted in a temperature controlled room (20°C) at a constant relative humidity (53 per cent). Healthy subjects (and patients) were unrestrained in their physical activities and eating habits in the daytime-active study from 0.5 hours post-radioaerosol inhalation and in all studies after the initial 6-hour period.

Smoking was forbidden for one hour prior to and for the first 6 hours after the radioaerosol inhalation in all studies. The onset of sleep was judged by observation and hypnotics were not administered.

Results

Healthy subjects

Ventilatory function (FEV_1, FVC, and PEFR) assessed one hour prior to radioaerosol inhalation was similar in the four studies and is shown in Table 2. The group mean alveolar deposition (AD) and initial radioaerosol distribution expressed as PI for each study are also shown in Table 2.

Alveolar deposition was similar in the four studies whereas mean PI ranged from 0.43 to 0.57 although differences between studies, once again, were not of statistical significance.

Table 2

Mean ± SE pulmonary function indices for 10 healthy subjects and 10 mild asthmatics on the days of their lung mucociliary clearance assessments

| | Healthy subjects | | | | Asthmatics | |
	Day-active	Day-supine	Night-awake	Night-asleep	Day-active	Night-asleep
Predicted FEV (per cent)	4.00±0.18	4.00±0.17	3.90±0.21	4.00±0.18	2. 70±0.38	2.56±0.35
Predicted FVC (per cent)	4.60±0.23	4.60±0.24	4.50±0.25	4.60±0.26	3. 96±0.44	3.75±0.38
Predicted PEFR (per cent)	515± 28	525±30	511± 31	519±30	402 ±47	389±38
Predicted $MMFR_{25-75}$(Per cent)	—	—	—	—	2.15 ±0.41	1.65±0.35
Predicted $\dot{V}_{max}$ 25 (Per cent)	—	—	—	—	0.82±0.16	0.70±0.15
Predicted $\dot{V}_{max}$ 50 (per cent)	—	—	—	—	2.10±0.38	1.75±0.34
AD	55±3	50±4	54±4	52± 6	43±5	39±6
PI	0.57±0.09	0.49±0.03	0.50±0.08	0.43±0.04	0.48±0.07	0.47±0.09

The mean period of sleep was 4 h 38 min (range: 3 h 30 min to 4 h 57 min). The mean time from radioaerosol inhalation to the onset of sleep was 1 h 18 min (range: 1 h 5 min to 2 h 0 min) and time of awakening 5 h 56 min (range: 5 h 15 min to 6 h 10 min).

Figure 1 shows the group mean tracheobronchial clearance curves against time for the four studies. These have been derived from whole lung clearance curves by correcting for AD, i.e. subtracting the 24-hour whole-lung retention values. The curves for the three awake studies are similar. However, during sleep there is marked retention of deposited radioaerosol. The group mean ($\pm$ SE) tracheobronchial clearances from 0 to 6 hours post-inhalation were similar: 81 ± 3, 83 ± 7 and 79 ± 6 per cent for the day-active, day-supine, and night-awake studies, respectively. On the other hand, for the night-asleep study the tracheobronchial clearance for the same period was only 42 ± 4 per cent and was significantly reduced ($P<0.01$) relative to each of the other three studies.

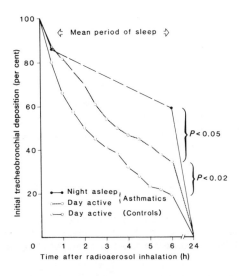

Fig. 1. Mean tracheobronchial mucociliary clearance curves for 10 healthy subjects measured during: (a) daytime-active; (b) daytime-supine; (c) nighttime-awake; and (d) nighttime-asleep.

Asthma patients

Ventilatory function: FEV_1, FVC, PEFR, $MMFR_{25-75}$, $\dot{V}_{max}25$, and $\dot{V}_{max}50$ assessed one hour prior to radioaerosol inhalation for the two studies is also shown in Table 2. There was no significant change from daytime to nighttime for large-airway function although there was a significant deterioration of small-airways function at night ($P<0.05$). The group mean AD and PI were similar for the two runs and are also shown in Table 2.

The mean period of sleep was 5 h 17 min (range: 4 h 43 min to 6 h 30 min). The mean time after radioaerosol inhalation to the onset of sleep was 48 min (range : 40 to 60 min) and time of awakening 6 h 03 min (range: 5 h 39 min to 7 h 10 min). Five patients had undisturbed periods of sleep, four patients woke up once, and the remaining one four times during the 'period of sleep'.

During the daytime-active runs three asthmatics coughed sputum (0.9, 1.2 and 9.0 g) whilst in the night-asleep only one asthmatic coughed 2.1 g of sputum.

Figure 2 shows the group mean tracheobronchial clearance curves against time for the day-active and night-asleep studies. Once again, the night-asleep curve is markedly reduced compared to the day-active curve. The group mean ($\pm$SE) tracheobronchial clearance values from 0 to 6 hours post-inhalation were: 65$\pm$9 and

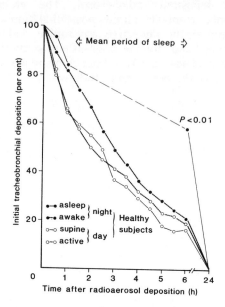

Fig. 2. *Mean tracheobronchial mucociliary clearance curves for 10 mild asthmatics measured during: (a) daytime-active; (b) nighttime asleep. For comparison purposes the mean daytime-active clearance curve is shown of 10 healthy subjects.*

41$\pm$11 per cent for the day-active and night-asleep, respectively ($P<0.05$). At six hours, there was a significant difference ($P<0.02$; unpaired Wilcoxon test) between the tracheobronchial clearance for asthmatic patients and the healthy subjects — both measured during the day-active studies. However, during sleep both groups achieved clearance rates which were similar to each other.

Discussion

These results indicate that normal physical activity, posture, and circadian rhythms have no effect on clearance of tracheobronchial secretions in health whereas sleep *per se* markedly reduces tracheobronchial mucociliary clearance both in healthy subjects and asthmatics.

Differences in the initial distribution of deposited radioaerosol within the lungs can result in differing clearance rates. For example, particles deposited in the proximal airways will generally be cleared faster than those deposited in the more distal ciliated airways due to their shorter transit path from deposition site to trachea. The partitioning of the deposited particles between the conducting/ciliated airways and alveolated regions was similar between runs, within the healthy subjects and asthmatics groups. PI was virtually the same in the asthmatic patients for the two studies. For the healthy subjects, however, PI was on average (but not statistically significantly so) less in the night-asleep study compared to the other three studies. This, if anything, should have resulted in a faster tracheobronchial mucociliary clearance during the night-asleep run. In the event the converse was found.

An increase in lung mucociliary clearance has been reported during exercise (briskly pedalling on a cycle ergometer for 20 min) both in healthy subjects (Wolff *et al*. 1977) and in patients with chronic bronchitis (Oldenburg *et al*. 1979). Eucapnic hyperventilation has also been reported to increase mucociliary clearance although to a lesser extent than exercise (Wolff *et al*. 1977). The mechanical effect of increased lung movement, mucus-gland hypersecretion from parasympathetic discharge, and ciliary stimulation by exercise-induced catecholamine release have been postulated as possible mechanisms for these observations (Wolff *et al*. 1977). In our studies, clearance during normal physical activity and rest (daytime-active vs. daytime-supine) were similar. It thus seems possible that the degree of physical activity or exercise is an important factor enhancing lung mucociliary clearance. The finding that posture (daytime-active vs. daytime-supine) had no effect on lung clearance in healthy subjects is in agreement with previous work (Friedman *et al*. 1977; Wong *et al*. 1977). Postural drainage however is an important aspect of chest physiotherapy capable of enhancing clearance in patients with copious secretions (Sutton *et al*. 1983).

The effect of circadian rhythm on lung mucociliary clearance has not to our knowledge previously been examined. From our studies on healthy subjects (daytime-supine vs. nighttime-awake) it appears to be unimportant.

The small difference likely to be encountered in ventilatory rate between nighttime-awake vs. nighttime-asleep runs (although not measured) would not be expected to account for the reduction in clearance observed during sleep with the healthy subjects and asthmatic patients.

One explanation for the stimulatory effect of severe exercise and inhibition by sleep could be that this most important defence mechanism of the lungs, namely mucociliary clearance, is under homeostatic control as exists for example with cardiac output, body temperature, and other metabolic processes. As a host defence mechanism, the mucociliary escalator is required to be continuously active in order to maintain a sterile tracheobronchial tree. However during sleep, deposition of inhaled particuiate matter on the conducting airways is probably reduced. The ambient surroundings are stable, the nose acts as an efficient filter under resting conditions (assuming nose breathing), and ventilation remains at a basal level. The host defence may not be unduly endangered therefore by a reduced mucociliary clearance during sleep in health whereas normal or increased action is necessary to ensure protection of the lung during physical activity and particularly so during exercise.

A homeostatic mechanism for the mucociliary escalator of the tracheobronchial tree has not been elucidated. Many pharmacological agents including cholinergic and adrenergic drugs can increase mucociliary action whereas anticholinergic and beta-adrenergic blocking agents can result in a retardation (Wanner 1977). This alteration in function can be brought about by changes in the quantity, biochemical content, and physical properties of pulmonary secretions and/or a direct effect on the ciliary beat frequency. On this basis homeostatis may be maintained by neurochumoral control via cholinergic and adrenergic mediators.

The finding of a reduced tracheobronchial daytime-active clearance in asthmatics relative to a comparable group (with regard to physical characteristics and tobacco consumption) of healthy subjects is in accord with our previous observations (Bateman *et al*. 1983). Airway plugging with mucus, in addition to oedema and smooth-muscle spasm, is an important pathological feature of asthma (Dunnill

1971). Impaired mucociliary clearance has been proposed as a cause for this mucus plugging both in asthmatics and non-asthmatics (Irwin and Thomas 1973). However the evidence linking abnormal mucus transport to airways obstruction is only indirect. Cochrane and colleagues (1977) found increases of 18 per cent in specific airway conductance and FEV_1, following the removal of copious pulmonary secretions in chronic bronchitis patients treated by physiotherapy. Gamsu et al. (1976) showed that delayed mucociliary clearance in patients following abdominal surgical procedures resulted in areas of mucus pooling within the lungs which were followed by subsequent atelectasis.

The delay in mucus transport seen in asthmatics during the day and particularly so during the night may contribute to airway obstruction and early-morning wheeze. However other diurnal variations may also be involved. Recent studies indicate that there is no significant change in adrenoceptor-mediated response in asthma at night (Barnes et al. 1981, 1982). Other possibilities are the effect of endogenous cortisol (Soutar et al. 1975) and catecholamine levels (Fairfax et al. 1980). It is worth noting that therapeutic agents such as oral aminophylline and beta sympathomimetics which are successful in abolishing nocturnal wheeze (Fairfax et al. 1980; Turner-Warwick 1977) have also been shown to enhance mucociliary clearance (Sutton et al. 1981) in addition to having bronchodilator properties. If this reduction in mucociliary clearance in asthmatics during sleep does contribute to the nocturnal asthma, then the administration of these drugs in sustained release form is further supported.

There are other implications of a reduced lung mucociliary clearance during sleep. If during sleep post-nasal drip reaches the tracheobronchial tree then it is likely to remain in situ overnight and thus spread infection as well as cause early-morning cough. If shiftworkers choose to sleep soon afterwards, then potentially any inhaled materials from the working environment may remain in the lungs for prolonged periods of time, predisposing them to occupational lung disease. Post-operative pneumonia and atelectasis may follow impairment of lung mucociliary clearance due to the post-operative medication (anticholinergic drugs), the type of anaesthetic gases used, lack of appropriate humidification, post-operative analgesics, and immobility (Gamsu et al. 1976; Barnes et al. 1981, 1982; Soutar et al. 1975; Fairfax et al. 1980; Turner-Warwick 1977; Sutton et al. 1981; Pavia and Thomson 1971) — sleep should now also be included in this list as a further possible contributor.

Finally, cigarette smoke is ciliostatic (Pavia et al. 1971); the last cigarette at night before going to sleep may well be the most harmful one since any inhaled carcinogens are likely to remain in situ for a prolonged period of time.

Conclusions

The effects of normal physical activity, posture, circadian rhythm, and sleep on tracheobronchial mucociliary clearance (T-B.M.C.) were assessed in a controlled, randomized, cross-over study involving 10 healthy subjects. In a further similar study the effect of sleep on T-B.M.C. was ascertained in a group of 10 mild but stable asthmatics. Lung mucociliary clearance was measured using an objective, noninvasive, radioaerosol technique. Simple physical activity (that corresponding to a normal working day), posture (i.e. erect vs. supine) and circadian rhythm (i.e. daytime vs. nighttime) were found to have no effect on lung mucociliary clearance. Sleep per se was found significantly to reduce T-B.M.C. by the same extent in healthy subjects as in asthmatics. These findings suggest that mucociliary function is under homeostatic control and that its reduction during sleep may contribute to early morning cough and expectoration or wheeze in patients with asthma.

Acknowledgements

The experimental work reported in this article was carried out with P.P. Sutton, J.R.M. Bateman, Nóirín F. Sheahan, J.E. Agnew and S.W. Clarke whom I thank for their advice and useful suggestions whilst preparing this manuscript. The figures were drawn by Michelle Clay.

References

Barnes, P.J., Brown, M.J., Silverman, M., and Dollery, C.T. (1981). *Thorax* **36**, 435.
Barnes, P.J., Fitzgerald, G.A., and Dollery, C.T. (1982). *Clin. Sci.* **62**, 349.
Bateman, J.R.M., Clarke, S.W., Pavia, D. and Sheahan, N.F. (1978) *a*). *J. Physicol.* **284**, 55P.
Bateman, J.R.M., Pavia, D., and Clarke, S.W. (1978) *b*). *Clin. Sci. mol. Med.* **55**, 523.
Bateman, J.R.M., Pavia, D., Sheahan, N.F., Agnew, J.E., and Clarke, S.W. (1983). *Thorax* **38**, 463.
Cammer, P. and Philipson, K. (1978). *Arch. environ. Hlth.* **36**, 181.
Catterall, J.R., Calverley, P.M.A., Brezinova, V., Douglas, N.J., Brash, H.M., Shapiro, C.M. and Flenley, D.C. (1982). *Lancet* **i**, 301.
Clark, T.J.H. and Hetzel, M.R. (1977). *Br. J. Dis. Chest.* **71**, 87.
Cochrane, G.M. and Clarke, T.J.H. (1975). *Thorax* **30**, 300.
Cochrane, G.M., Webber, B.A. and Clarke, S.W. (1977). *Br. med. J.* **2**, 1181.
Cotes, J.E. (1975).*Lung function*, 3rd ed. Blackwell Scientific Publications (Oxford).
Dawson, H., Douglas, R.B., Pavia, D., Reeves, E., Short, M.D., and Thomson, M.L.(1971). *Phys. Med. Biol.* **16**, 691.
Dunnill, M.S. (1971). In *Identification of asthma* (ed. R. Porter. and J. Birch), CIBA Foundation Study Group No. 38, Churchill Livingstone, Edinburgh & London.
Fairfax, A.J., McNabb, W.R. Davies, H.J., and Spiro, S.G. (1980). *Thorax* **35**, 526.
Few, J.D., Short, M.D., and Thomson, M.L. (1970). *Radiochem. Radioanal. Lett.* **5**, 275.
Friedman, M., Stott, F.D., Poole, D.O., Dougherty, R., Chapman, G.H., Watson, M., and Sackner, M.A. (1977). *Am. Rev. resp. Dis.* **115**, 67.
Gamsu, G., Singer, M.M., Vincent, H.H., Berry, S. and Nadel, J.A. (1976). *Am. Rev. resp. Dis.* **114**, 673.
Goodman, R.M., Yergin, B.M., Landa, J.F., Golinvaux, M.H., and Sackner, M.A. (1978). *Am. Rev. resp. Dis.* **117**, 205.
Guillerm, R., Badre, R., Hee, J., and Pastore, R. (1966). *J. Physiol.*, (*Paris*) **58**, 228.
Hetzel, M.R., Clark, T.J.H., and Branthwaite, M.A.(1977). *Br. med. J.* **1**, 808.
Hirsch, J.A., Tokayer, J.L., Robinson, M.J., and Sackner, M.A. (1975). *J. appl. Physiol.* **39**, 242.
Irwin, R.S. and Thomas, H.M. (1973). *Am. Rev. resp. Dis.***108**, 985.
Knudson, R.J., Slatin, R.C., Lebowitz, M.D., and Burrows, B. (1976). *Am. Rev. resp. Dis.* **113**, 587.
Lourenço, R.V., Klimek, M.F., and Borowski, C.J. (1971). *J. clin. Invest.* **50**, 1411.
Oldenburg, F.A., Dolovich, M.B., Montgomery, J.M., and Newhouse, M.T. (1979). *Am. Rev. resp. Dis.* **120**, 739.
Pavia, D., Bateman, J.R.M., and Clarke, S.W. (1980). *Bull. Eur. Physiopath. Resp.* **16**, 335.
Pavia, D., Sutton, P.P., Agnew, J.E., Lopez-Vidriero, M.T., Newman, S.P., and Clarke, S.W. (1983). *Eur. J. resp. Dis.* **64** (Suppl. 127), 41.
Pavia, D., Sutton P.P., Lopez-Vidriero, M.T., Agnew, J.E., and Clarke, S.W. (1983). *Eur. J. resp. Dis.* **64** (suppl. 128), 304.
Pavia, D. and Thomson, M.L. (1971). *Lancet* **i**, 449.
Pavia, D., Thomson, M.L., and Pocock, S.J. (1971). *Nature* **231**, 325.
Puchelle, E., Zahm, Z-M. and Bertrand, A. (1979). *Scand. J. resp. Dis.* **60**, 307.
Soutar, C.A., Costello, J., Ijaduola, O., and Turner-Warwick, M. (1975). *Thorax* **30**, 436.

Sutton, P.P., Parker, R.A., Webber, B.A., Newman, S.P., Garland, N., Lopez-Vidriero, M.T., Pavia, D., and Clarke, S.W. (1983). *Eur. J. resp. Dis.* **64**, 62.

Sutton, P.P., Pavia, D., Bateman, J.R.M., and Clarke, S.W. (1981). *Chest* **80** (suppl.), 889.

Thomson, M.L. and Pavia, D. (1973). *Arch. environ. Hlth.* **26**, 86.

Turner-Warwick, M.T. (1977). *Br. J. Dis. Chest* **71**, 228.

Wanner, A. (1977). *Am. Rev. resp. Dis.* **116**, 73.

Wolff, R.K., Dolovich, M.B., Obminski, G., and Newhouse, M.T. (1977). *J. appl. Physiol.* **43**, 46.

Wong, J.W., Keens, T.G., Wannamaker, E.M., Douglas, P.T., Crozier, N., Levison, H., and Aspin, N. (1977). *Paediatrics* **60**, 146.

Discussion

Professor D.C. Flenley

Were the asthmatic and the normal subjects age-matched?

Dr D. Pavia

The healthy subjects had a mean age of 30 and the asthmatics had a mean age of 34 years.

Dr G. Laszlo

Is there any correlation between nocturnal asthma and morning sputum?

Professor D.C. Flenley

Cough in children is thought to be an asthmatic symptom because it gets better with bronchodilators. There is a current study in Edinburgh recording cough at night in children in their own homes and with a placebo control to see if this is true.

Dr M. Silverman

A survey from Newcastle which was published in the *British Medical Journal* last year showed that children who have nocturnal cough have a much greater bronchial responsiveness than children who don't, so that there is probably some objective relationship between nocturnal cough and asthma in children.

Professor T.J. Clark

Do you have any observations about changes of mucociliary clearance in individual asthmatics with changes in their asthmatic state?

Dr D. Pavia

We have done a study on patients admitted to hospital with status asthmaticus who were able to reach our research laboratory within two days of admission, where clearance was reduced. Clearance was then measured a week or so after admission before being sent home and subsequently two to three months after the initial attack; there was no change in the degree of impairment in clearance, which seemed to last for the duration of time that we examined the patients.

Dulfano and colleagues suggested that there is a 'ciliary inhibitory factor' of molecular weight of 6000–8000 in the sputum of asthmatic patients. When placed on human airway cilia it reduces ciliatory beat frequency, and seems to be related to the degree of exacerbation of the asthmatic attack.

Dr C.K. Connolly

Were the abnormalities present in all asthmatics and, if not, was there any relationship either to the age of the subject or the length of time the patient had had asthma? I ask this because there is a strong suggestion that chronic airway obstruction develops over the years in patients whom one would diagnose as atopic asthmatics.

Dr D. Pavia

We have no idea about the relationship in this small group between severity of asthma and impairment. From other studies in patients with chronic bronchitis there is no evidence that the degree of impairment in mucociliary clearance is correlated with the degree of impairment of lung function. Two previous studies have shown that age impairs mucociliary clearance but from our unpublished data we have not been able to confirm this in healthy subjects.

Dr D. Reid

I presume that the reduction in clearance in healthy patients at night is due to the reduction in metabolic function at night.

Dr D. Pavia

We do not know why mucociliary clearance is impaired at night. There may be a reduction in ciliary beat frequency, possibly due to a variation in circulation because of cooling, but this is only a hypothesis.

Circadian Rhythms: Their Physiology and Relevance to Asthma

D.S. MINORS

Department of Physiology, University of Manchester, Manchester M13 9PT, UK

Rhythmicity — a general principle

A ubiquitous feature of Nature is that of rhythmicity. Such rhythms are most obvious in our environment; thus, there are the regular oscillators, such as the day-to-night changes in light intensity and ambient temperature, associated with the solar day and the regular annual changes through the seasons to be found in all but equatorial regions. In addition, however, rhythmicity is also a general principle in biology and rhythms can be observed across phylogeny (Ashchoff 1963; Cloudsley-Thompson 1980; Palmer 1976). Though biological rhythms which have a short period (the period of a rhythm is the time to complete one cycle), such as the heart beat and gastric slow wave, have been observed and documented for many years, less obvious are rhythms which oscillate infrequently and can only be detected if observations are made over many days or months. Most of these rhythms which have a long period are synchronized to some environmental rhythmicity. Thus, those species, such as the fiddler crab, which inhabit the shorelines are synchronized to the lunar day as a result of the tides. For most species, however, the most obvious environmental changes are those associated with the solar day. Correspondingly, it is found that many aspects of a plant's or animal's physiology and biochemistry oscillate with a period of 24 hours — the length of the solar day. Such rhythms are termed circadian (from the latin *circa*: about; *dies*: a day) and this term encompasses those rhythms with a period in the range 21–28 hours (Halberg 1959). Thus, although the general principles of homeostasis still hold, it must be realized that there is a temporal order to many aspects of a plant's or animal's physiology.

Circadian rhythms have been described at all levels of organisation — from whole organisms, through organs, to individual cells, in practically every species studied so far. In man, too, these rhythms are dominant. Figure 1 shows the normal circadian rhythm found in deep body temperature, plasma 11-hydroxycorticosteroid concentration, blood pressure, and urinary excretion of potassium in a healthy human subject. Most other aspects of human physiology likewise show a clear circadian variation and have been reviewed elsewhere (Minors and Waterhouse 1981; Moore-Ede *et al*. 1982). Indeed, today it is a greater challenge to demonstrate a variable which does not display circadian variation!

The role of these circadian rhythms is to permit an organism to fit better into its environment (Daan and Aschoff 1982). Thus, for example, it can be seen in Fig. 1

that deep body temperature and the secretion of the glucocorticoids begin to rise in advance of the habitual waking time. In this way the body is prepared for the rigours and stresses of the next day. The existence of circadian rhythms thus enable an

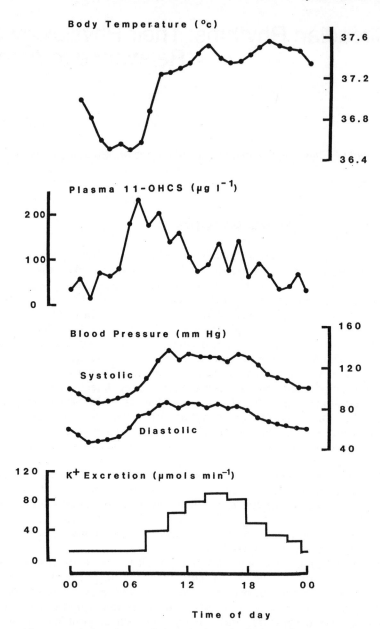

Fig. 1. The normal circadian variations in deep body (rectal) temperature, plasma 11-hydroxycorticosteroids, blood pressure, and urinary excretion of potassium in a healthy subject. (Unpublished data of Minors.)

animal to anticipate 24-hour environmental changes and bring about appropriate responses. An analogy more familiar to the physiologist is the advantage gained by the use of cutaneous thermoreceptors through which future changes in deep body temperature can be estimated and acted upon; thus the efficiency of the thermoregulatory mechanisms is optimized.

The endogeneity of rhythms

When observed in normal, healthy individuals, circadian rhythms show remarkable stability; their period is exactly 24 hours. Although the waveform and/or phase (position in time) of a circadian rhythm may vary slightly between individuals, in a given individual it is usually quite stable.

In view of the stability of circadian rhythms and their synchronisation to the solar day, it is tempting to ascribe them to a passive response of the body to its rhythmic environment. Thus, in humans, it might be predicted that, for example, body temperature and blood pressure will show higher values during the daytime than during the night since our social behaviour is based upon diurnal work and wakefulness and nocturnal rest and sleep. However, as indicated above, these variables show rises before wakefulness indicating that these bodily rhythms cannot solely be a passive response of the body. Furthermore, such rhythms will continue even if an individual is kept in constant environmental conditions. Figure 2 shows the mean body temperature rhythm measured in a group of eight subjects who remained

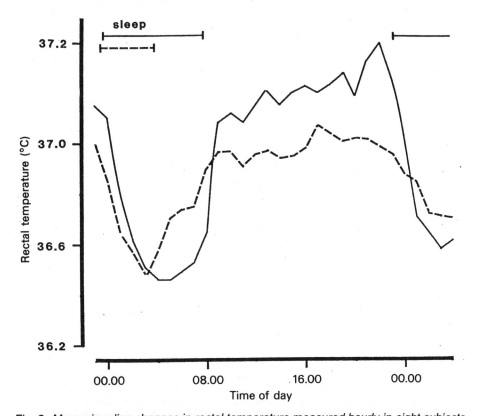

Fig. 2. Mean circadian changes in rectal temperature measured hourly in eight subjects living a normal nychthemeral existance (solid line) and in the same subjects awoken at 04.00 and spending the subsequent 24 hours awake in constant conditions. (From Minors and Waterhouse (1981), Fig. 2.2.)

awake and sedentary for 24 hours in a soundproofed constantly-lit room maintained at a constant temperature and humidity. It can be seen that, despite the constant conditions, the rhythm in body temperature is still evident. Such evidence leads to the conclusion that circadian rhythms must be controlled by some internal oscillator. This endogenous timing mechanism is metaphorically referred to as the 'biological clock'.

Although an overt rhythm may be controlled by an endogenous oscillator, this is not to say that rhythms in our environment and other external rhythms are without effect. Thus, in Fig. 2 it can been seen that normal diurnal activity elevates body temperature and nocturnal sleep decreases it. Furthermore, it has been shown that the diminution of body temperature by sleep is itself subject to circadian variation, with greater decrements in temperature being seen with nocturnal sleep than with sleep diurnally (Mills *et al.* 1978*a*). Such direct effects of external influences on circadian rhythms are referred to as the exogenous component or masking effect.

Further evidence for a component of overt circadian rhythms being endogenous in nature is gained from the behaviour of rhythms in animals kept in constant conditions for many days or months. Under such conditions the rhythms continue oscillations, but with a period deviating from an exact 24 hours — the rhythms are said to be 'free-running' (Bruce and Pittendrigh 1957). The exact period of such free-running rhythms depends upon the species under investigation, but it always deviates from an exact 24 hours. It is for this reason that these rhythms are described as *circa*dian — the period is *about* a day. Since the period of free-running rhythms deviates from that of the solar day, this is strong evidence for the endogeneity of rhythms. Furthermore, there seems a genetic basis for this endogeneity since free-

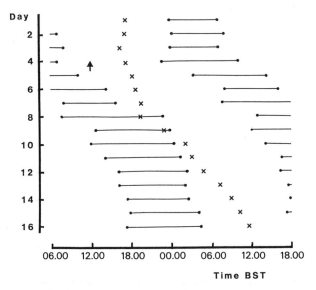

Fig. 3. *Circadian changes in sleep and wakefulness and body temperature in a free-running experiment performed on a human subject in an isolation chamber. Bars represent the time of sleep on successive days from above downwards; X, daily time of maximum of body temperature. For the first three days of the experiment the subject was provided with a clock which registered correct time. On day 4, at the point indicated by the arrow, the clock was removed and rhythms free-ran with a period in excess of 24 hours.* (Data of Mills *et al.* (1974).

running rhythms can be observed in mice exposed for five successive generations to constant conditions (Aschoff 1960).

The presence of an endogenous clock with an inherent period deviating from an exact 24 hours has also been established in humans by isolating subjects from time cues. The first such experiment was performed by Aschoff and Wever (1962) using a converted cellar. Since this early experiment many others have been performed (Mills *et al*. 1974; Wever 1979; Czeisler 1978; Czeisler *et al*. 1980). Often these experiments have been performed in specially constructed isolation units where subjects can be isolated from not only the more obvious cues as to the time of day, such as the alternation of light and dark, but also from sound, ground-borne vibrations, and fluctuations in mains electrical voltage — all of which may be used to assess the time of day. An example of free-running rhythms in a human subject is shown in Fig. 3; it can be seen that, following the initial control period during which a 24-hour clock was provided when the clock was removed and the subject allowed to free-run, the times of sleep and of maximum body temperature became later on each successive day. This indicates the continued oscillation of the rhythms of sleep and wakefulness and of body temperature with a period in excess of 24 hours, though the subject was quite unaware of this. By far the largest series of free-running experiments on humans has been performed in Germany (Wever 1979) in which a study of 152 subjects has yielded an average free-running period of 25.0 ± 0.49 hours.

Entrainment of rhythms

From the foregoing, it is obvious that the inherent period of the endogenous clock controlling circadian rhythms in man is greater than 24 hours. For the rhythms controlled by such a clock to be advantageous and allow us to fit better into our 24-hour environment, it is evident that the inherent clock must be adjusted (entrained) to run with a period of 24 hours. Indeed, it is found that, when a rhythm is measured in an individual living in normal conditions, its period is exactly 24 hours. Thus, although not a totally appropriate analogy, the biological clock has been likened to a watch which runs slow but can be adjusted to register correct time.

The entrainment of the endogenous clock to an exact 24 hours is believed to be achieved by rhythmic influences in our environment which have a period of exactly 24 hours. Such an influence is termed a 'zeitgeber' (Aschoff 1954) — the German word meaning time-giver — or a 'synchroniser' (Halberg *et al*. 1954). Although there are many potential zeitgebers in our environment, such as the day-to-night swings of air temperature, the most obvious daily change is the alternation between light and dark. It is the 24 hour light–dark cycle which has shown to be the most important zeitgeber in most mammals. Only in man has the role of the daily light–dark cycle as a zeitgeber been a matter of some dispute. Thus, Wever (1970, 1979) has argued that the light–dark cycle is a rather weak zeitgeber in man, since he demonstrated free-running rhythms in subjects studied in an isolation chamber with an imposed 24-hour light–dark cycle. However, the subjects in these experiments were free to use auxiliary lighting during the period when the main room lights were switched off. Thus there was no real need to make use of the rhythmic information provided by the imposed light–dark cycle. More recently, in experiments performed by Czeisler and his colleagues (1981) in which a strict light–dark cycle was imposed with no auxiliary lighting, it was shown that subjects were entrained by the light–dark cycle. In these experiments the role of the light-dark cycle would seem clear enough but human behavioural patterns would dictate that it would be difficult not to comply — what else could be done in a period of eight hours of complete darkness other than to go to bed and sleep!

It is believed by the present author that the alternation of sleep and wakefulness related to our social life is the most important zeitgeber in man. That is, normal domestic and business activities take place during the daytime and so we are awake during these hours; we know that a certain amount of sleep is required to prepare for the rigours of the next day and this directs our time of retiring to bed. Once the sleep–wakefulness cycle has been established, all other potential zeitgebers are manipulated by us to coincide with this cycle (for example during the winter evenings we use artificial lighting to be able to continue our leisure activities).

Central mechanisms controlling circadian rhythms

Ever since the realization that circadian rhythms must be driven by some endogenous oscillator, it has been speculated that the obvious site for the biological

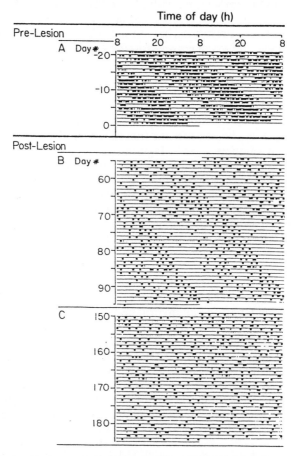

Fig. 4. Drinking rhythm in a squirrel monkey before (A) and after (B, C) a histologically verified total SCN lesion. Throughout, the monkey was kept in constant conditions. Before the lesion (A) a free-running rhythm with a period of approximately 25 hours is seen. After the lesion (B) the rhythm gradually decays eventually becoming arrhythmic (C). (From Moore-Ede et al. (1982) Fig. 4.16)

clock would be in the central nervous system. It was not until the many exhaustive studies of Richter in 1967, however, that the major clue to the siting of the biological clock in mammals was obtained. Richter placed hundreds of lesions in various parts of the brain of blinded rats and found that only when lesions were placed in an area of the ventral hypothalamus were the drinking, feeding, and activity rhythms in these animals lost.

Since this pioneering study, the circadian oscillator has been located in the suprachiasmatic nuclei (SCN), two small groups of cells in the ventral hypothalamus just dorsal to the optic chiasm. Thus, the loss of circadian rhythms in drinking and activity in hamsters (Stephan and Zucker 1972) and of the adrenal corticosterone rhythm in rats (Moore and Eichler 1972) following ablation of the SCN were first reported. Numerous other studies since these have confirmed the loss of rhythmicity following SCN lesions and have been severally reviewed (Moore 1979*a, b*, 1983; Rusak 1977; Rusak and Zucker 1979; Block and Page 1978; Raisman and Brown-Grant 1977). An example of the ultimate breakdown of rhythms following SCN ablation is shown in Fig. 4 which shows the gradual decay of the drinking rhythm in the squirrel monkey following SCN ablation.

The loss of rhythmicity following SCN ablation does not in itself indicate that the SCN is the site of the circadian oscillator. Rather, it might only indicate that the SCN forms some link between an oscillator elsewhere in the CNS and the final overt appearance of rhythms. Further evidence that the SCN functions as a circadian oscillator is provided by the following evidence:–

1. The electrophysiological activity of hypothalamic 'islands' (including the SCN), surgically isolated from surrounding brain structures, shows circadian variation with higher daytime activity than nighttime activity (Inouye and Kawamura 1979).
2. Continuing circadian variation in the electrophysiological activity of *in vitro* slices of hypothalamic tissue containing the SCN have been observed (Green and Gillette 1982; Groos and Hendriks 1982; Groos *et al.* 1983).
3. By measuring the rate of uptake glucose using the 2-deoxyglucose method, a rhythm in the metabolic activity of the SCN *in vivo* has been demonstrated (Schwartz and Gainer 1977; Schwartz *et al.* 1980).
4. Electrical stimulation of the SCN has been shown to cause changes in the period of, and phase shifts in, free-running circadian rhythms (Rusak and Groos 1982).
5. Even before the demonstration of the loss of rhythmicity following SCN ablation, a direct monosynaptic connection, the retinohypothalamic tract, between the retina and SCN in the rat was demonstrated (Moore and Lenn 1972); this has been confirmed in many more species since (see Moore (1983) for review). This tract forms the anatomical basis for the entrainment of the circadian oscillator by light–dark cycles.

The experiments performed above, of course, have not been performed in humans. It is relevant to note, however, a group of neurones homologous to the SCN of lower species has been shown histologically in humans (Lydic *et al.* 1980). The control of circadian rhythms in man and primates, however, seems more complex than in lower species. Thus, there is growing evidence that rhythms in man and primates are controlled by two oscillators. Evidence for this first came from the behaviour of rhythms in free-running experiments performed by Aschoff's group on humans (summarized by Wever 1979). They found that, in about one-third of subjects studied in free-running experiments, the phenomenon of spontaneous internal desynchronization was observed. An example of this phenomenon is shown in Fig. 5. Initially, on days 1–14, before internal desynchronization occurred, the rhythm of sleep and wakefulness and of body temperature free-ran with an identical period (25.7 hours) so that there was a constant phase relationship between the two rhythms. About day 15, however, internal desynchronization between the sleep–

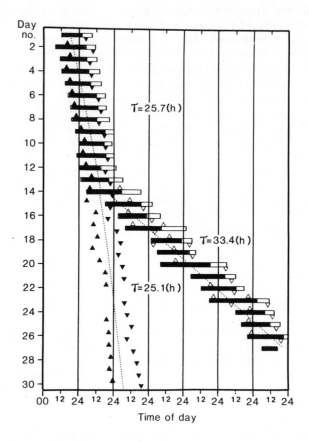

Fig. 5. Circadian rhythms of sleep and wakefulness (white and black bars respectively) and of rectal temperature (▼ maxima, ▲ minima) in a subject in temporal isolation. Successive days are plotted from above downwards. From days 1 through 14 the subject is internally synchronized with the two rhythms showing similar periods (25.7 hours). At day 15 spontaneous desynchronization takes place so that thereafter the two rhythms show different periods (rectal temperature 25.1 hours; sleep – wakefulness 33.4 hours). Open triangles show temporally corrected positions of temperature, maxima and minima represented by corresponding black triangles. (From Wever (1975), Fig. 7.)

wakefulness cycle and the rhythm of body temperature took place, with the sleep–wakefulness cycle lengthening to a period of 33.4 hours whilst the body temperature rhythm shortened its period slightly to 25.1 hours. A similar phenomenon has also been observed in the squirrel monkey (Sulzman *et al.* 1977). Subsequently, it has been shown, both in man and the squirrel monkey, that, when internal desynchronization takes place, overt rhythms tend to cluster in two groups; one group showing a predominant period the same as the sleep–wakefulness rhythm and the other following the period of the temperature rhythm (Moore-Ede *et al.* 1982; Wever 1975, 1979; Czeisler 1978; Sulzman *et al.* 1977; Weitzman *et al.* 1979). This is strong evidence that, in man and primates, circadian rhythms are controlled by two oscillators which Moore-Ede (1983; Moore-Ede *et al.* 1982) has termed 'X' (body-temperature driving) and 'Y' (sleep–wakefulness driving) and which Wever (1975) has termed Type I (body-temperature driving) and Type II (sleep-wakefulness driving oscillator). Under normal conditions, the two oscillators are coupled to one another so that any overt rhythm results from the activities of both. Under conditions of internal desynchronization, however, they become dissociated and overt rhythms become desynchronized following the activity of the oscillator by which they are dominantly controlled. As shown in Fig. 5, since the period of rhythms, before internal desynchronization takes place, is closer to the period of the temperature rhythm after desynchronization, it is further argued that the X or Type I oscillator is much stronger (4–8 times) than the Y or Type II oscillator.

The question remains as to whether the SCN corresponds to X (Type I) or Y (Type II) oscillator. Recent experiments on the rhesus (Mills *et al.* 1978 *b*) and squirrel monkeys (Elliott *et al.* 1972) have shown that not all rhythms disappear after lesion of the SCN in these species. Rather, feeding, activity, and drinking (Fig. 4) rhythms were disrupted, suggesting that the Y (Type II) oscillator lies within the SCN. On the other hand, the deep body temperature rhythm in the squirrel monkey and the rhythm of cortisol in the rhesus monkey (a rhythm which usually follows the temperature rhythm) were not disrupted, suggesting that the X (Type I) oscillator lies outside the SCN.

The stability of rhythms

Although zeitgebers may entrain the circadian oscillator from its inherent period of about 25 hours in humans to an exact 24 hours, the range of entrainment of the circadian rhythms is very narrow, particularly those rhythms controlled by the X (Type I) oscillator. Typically, these rhythms may only be entrained by zeitgebers with periods in the range of approximately 23 to 27 hours.

The extreme stability of the biological clock has presented several problems to modern man. Thus, for example, the human circadian system is unable to undergo large, rapid phase-shifts (Mills *et al.* 1978 *b*; Elliott *et al.* 1972; Aschoff *et al.* 1975; Klein and Wegmann 1979). This has led to the phenomenon of 'jet-lag syndrome' following transmeridional flights and results from the circadian system being unable to shift its phase rapidly in accord with the change in external time; as a result there is a temporary mismatch between internal and external time which it is thought results in the ill-assorted group of symptoms collectively known as jet-lag syndrome. The adaptation of the human circadian system to time-zone shifts is reviewed in Minors and Waterhouse (1981), Chapter 9.

The other circumstance in which possession of an endogenous oscillator has proved to be disadvantageous in man is when we attempt to do shift work, particularly the night shift. The reason for this is that the individual working at night (and therefore sleeping during the day) is living at odds with natural zeitgebers and the rest of society. As a result he is able to shift his rhythms appropriate to his nocturnal activity only with considerable difficulty. This results in a feeling of fatigue during the waking period and a loss of sleep. Thus, the length of diurnal sleep is usually shorter than that in the same worker sleeping at night (see Rutenzfranz *et al.* 1976, for example). In addition, the inappropriate phasing of the worker's rhythms gives rise to malaise, particularly disorders of the gastrointestinal tract, often reported by shift workers (Harrington 1978). With continued time on the night shift, the worker's rhythms do begin to phase-shift, but any adaptation gained during the working week is often rapidly lost during days off, when the worker usually reverts to diurnal activity. Thus, at the beginning of the next working week adaptation must start afresh. The problems associated with shift work are reviewed in Minors and Waterhouse (1981), Chapter 10.

Implications of circadian rhythms to asthma

As might be predicted from the observation that most physiological variables exhibit circadian variation, so too pathophysiology is subject to circadian variation. At its extreme this can be seen by the circadian variation in mortality (Fig. 6) with two-thirds of deaths occurring between 4 a.m. and 11 a.m. It must be admitted, however, that the factors responsible for this rhythm have not been established.

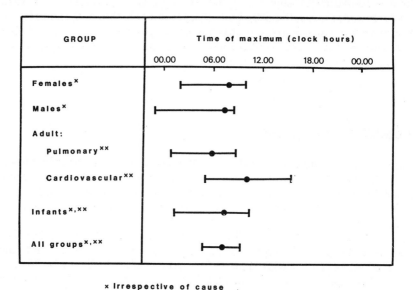

Fig. 6. *Circadian variation in mortality derived from a study of 400 000 deaths.* ● *time of peak, bars, 95 per cent confidence interval. Peak mortality is found in the hours between* 04.00 *and* 11.00 *irrespective of cause, age, or sex. (Data of Smolensky et al. (1972).*

At a lesser extreme, there are other pathophysiological conditions which show circadian variation in their occurrence and which may be explained, at least in part, by increased susceptibility due to normal circadian variation. A clear example of this is the finding of nocturnal and early morning asthma. As early as the third century A.D. it was realized that the dyspnoea of asthma was exacerbated during the normal times of sleep (Adams 1856). Since that time many others have confirmed that dyspnoea is maximal nocturnally or during the early morning (Reinberg *et al.* 1977; Prevost *et al.* 1980; Hetzel and Clark 1978; Gervais *et al.* 1978; Barnes *et al.* 1980; Reindl *et al.* 1969; Smolensky *et al.* 1981 for example). Traditionally, the nocturnal exacerbation of dyspnoea in asthmatics has been related to external (exogenous) factors, such as an increased exposure to antigens in, for example, bedding and the pulmonary changes associated with the adoption of the supine posture. Though these factors undoubtedly play a role, the nocturnal exacerbation of dyspnoea must owe part of its origin also to endogenous circadian variation of several physiological variables which have a phase so as to make an asthmatic attack more likely during the night or early morning. These rhythms have been summarized by Smolensky *et al.* (1977) and are shown in Fig. 7, taken from their paper. The figure shows the times at

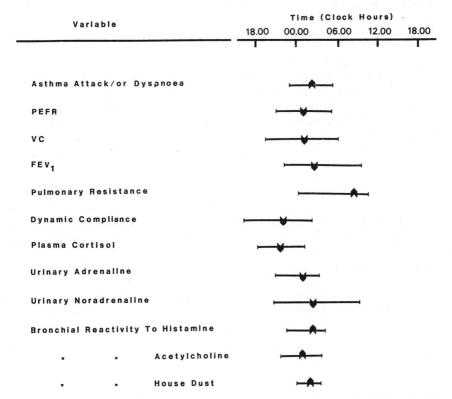

Fig. 7. *Circadian variations in factors predisposing to asthmatic attacks. Upward-pointing arrows indicate the time of maximum (in those variables for which high values exacerbate dyspnoea) and downwards-pointing arrows indicate the time of minimum (in those variables for which low values exacerbate dyspnoea). Horizontal bars represent the 95 per cent confidence intervals. (From Smolenksy et al. Fig. 5)*

which several variables likely to exacerbate dyspnoea reach a maximum (in the case of those variables where high values worsen dyspnoea) or a minimum (when low values are likely to worsen dyspnoea).

Thus,

1. Airway resistance, assessed both by PEFR (Reinberg *et al.* 1977; Prevost *et al.*

1980; Hetzel and Clark 1978; Gervais *et al.* 1978; Barnes *et al.* 1980; Reindl *et al.* 1969) and FEV (Barnes *et al.* 1980; Smolensky *et al.* 1977), has been found to be at a minimum about the usual time of waking. Though this rhythm is normally of small amplitude in healthy individuals (Smolensky *et al.* 1977; Gaultier *et al.* 1977), the amplitude and mean are elevated in asthmatics (Hetzel and Clark 1978; Smolensky *et al.* 1977).

2. A possible explanation for this rhythm in airway resistance is rhythmicity in the autonomic nervous system. Thus, minimum sympathetic activity as assessed by urinary or circulating adrenaline is found in the small hours (Minors and Waterhouse 1981; Barnes *et al.* 1980).

3. Histamine release reaches a maximum in the small hours (Barnes *et al.* 1980). In part this may, in turn, be explained by the normal rhythm in cortisol secretion which shows a minimum around midnight.

4. There are clear circadian variations in bronchial reactivity to histamine, acetylcholine, and house dust (Smolensky *et al.* 1981).

These factors will be discussed in further detail in future papers.

Not only do circadian rhythms have implications for the diagnosis and severity of symptoms of asthma but also further implications come from the observation that the pharmacology of many drugs is not invariate with time of day. This field, termed chronopharmacology, has been extensively investigated recently and numerous symposia and reviews have been devoted to this subject. Clear reviews of this topic can be found in Reinberg *et al.* (1981) and Reinberg and Smolensky (1982).

The time dependence of a drug can be considered in three ways.

1. *Chronesthesy*. This is a measure of rhythmic changes of the susceptibility of a system to a given dose of drug at different times of the nycthemeron. In general, it results from rhythmic changes in the quantity of receptors available. Thus, for example, bronchial reactivity to several substances including histamine, synthetic corticosteroids, and bronchodilators (including several ß-adrenoceptor agonists, theophylline, and vagolytic substances) shows circadian variation (Smolensky *et al.* 1981).

2. *Chronopharmacokinetics*. This is a measure of rhythmic changes in the time course of the concentration of a drug after administration at different times of the nycthemeron and results from rhythmic changes in the metabolism and/or excretion of the drug. It is becoming apparent that many of the drugs used in the treatment of asthma show circadian variation in their pharmacokinetics (see Smolensky *et al.* (1981) and Reinberg and Smolensky (1982) for a review of the literature).

3. *Chronergy*. This is defined as rhythmic changes in the effectiveness of the drug upon the system as a whole at different times of the nycthemeron. It includes both the therapeutic effect (chronoeffectiveness) and the toxic, side-effect (chronotoxicity). The chronergy of a drug is dependent, in turn, upon the chronesthesy of the target organ and the chronopharmacokinetics of the drug. By way of an example, Fig. 8 shows the circadian changes in PEFR in an asthmatic patient administered the synthetic corticosteroid Dutimelan® on two regimens. It can be seen that when administered at 08.00 and 15.00 the mean PEFR was greater than when administered at 15.00 and 20.00; in particular the nocturnal dip in PEFR was significantly reduced by the 08.00–15.00 treatment.

It is evident from the foregoing that, in the case of the asthmatic, not only should the type of drug used for treatment be considered but also, by considering the chronopharmacology of the drug, the efficiency of treatment may be optimised. The fact that circadian periodicities contribute to the predisposition of asthmatic attacks, together with the demonstrated chronopharmacology of several drugs, implies the need for further investigation of the chronobiology of

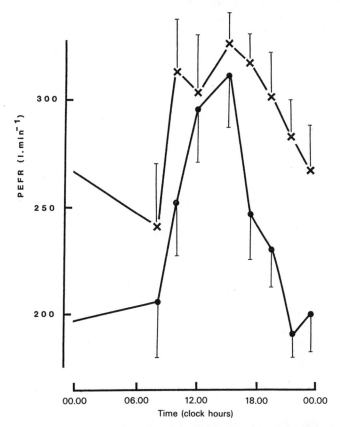

Fig. 8. Circadian variations in PEFR in a 30-year-old female asthmatic treated with Dutimelan ® on two regimens. In the first (x) a pill containing 7 mg of prednisolone acetate + 4 mg prednisolone alcohol was taken at 08.00 and a pill containing 3 mg of prednisolone alcohol + 15 mg of cortisone acetate was taken at 15.00. In the second treatment regimen ● the pill containing the prednisolone acetate – alcohol mixture was taken at 20.00 and the prednisolone – cortisone mixture at 15.00. Points represent mean values from measurements over eight days + or − 1 SE. Note the nocturnal dip is less and the mean higher with the prednisolone acetate – alcohol mixture taken at 08.00. (From Reinberg et al. (1983, Fig. 2.)

new drugs used in the treatment of asthma, as well as to re-evaluate and improve the efficiency of existing drugs by taking account of the time-dependent action of them. Thus modern medicine should ask not only how to treat but also *when* to treat so as to achieve maximal therapeutic effects with minimal toxic effects.

References

Adams, F. (1856). *The extant works of Aretaeus, the Cappadocian*. Sydenham Society, London.
Aschoff, J. (1954). *Naturwissenschaften* **41**, 49.

Aschoff, J. (1960). *Cold Spring Harbor Symp. quant. Biol.* **25**, 11.
Aschoff, J. (1963). *Ann. Rev. Physiol.* **25**, 581.
Aschoff, J., Hoffmann, K., Pohl, H., and Wever, R. (1975). *Chronobiologia* **2**, 23.
Aschoff, J. and Wever, R. (1962). Spontanperiodik des Menschen bei Ausschluss aller Zeitgeber. *Naturwissenschaften* **49**, 337.
Barnes, P., Fitzgerald, G., Brown, M., and Dollery, C. (1980). *New Engl. J. Med.* **303**, 263.
Block, G.D. and Page, T.L. (1978). *Ann. Rev. Neurosci.* **1**, 19–34.
Bruce, V.G. and Pittendrigh, C.S. (1957). *Am. Naturalist* **91**, 179–95.
Cloudsley-Thompson, J.L. (1980) *Biological clocks. Their functions in nature.* Weidenfeld and Nicolson, London.
Czeisler, C.A. (1978). Ph.D. thesis, Stanford University.
Czeisler, C.A., Richardson, G.S., Zimmerman, J.C., Moore-Ede, M.C. and Weitzman, E.D. (1981). *Photochem. Photobiol.* **34**, 239.
Czeisler, C.A., Weitzman, E.D., Moore-Ede, M.C., Zimmerman, J.C., and Knauer, R.S. (1980). Human sleep: its duration and organization depend on its circadian phase. *Science* **210**, 1264.
Daan, S. and Aschoff, J. (1982). In *Vertebrate circadian systems* (ed. J. Aschoff, S. Daan, and G.A. Groos), p.305. Springer-Verlag, New York.
Elliott, A.L., Mills, J.N., Minors, D.S., and Waterhouse, J.M. (1972). *J. Physiol.* **221**, 227–57.
Gaultier, C., Reinberg, A., and Girard, F. (1977). *Resp. Physiol.* **31**, 169–82.
Gervais, P., Reinberg, A., Fraboulet, G., Abulker, C., Vignaud, D., and Delcourt, M.E.R. (1978). In *Chronopharmacology* (ed. A. Reinberg and F. Halberg), p.203. Pergamon Press, Oxford.
Green, D.J. and Gillette, R. (1982). *Brain Res.* **245**, 198.
Groos, G. and Hendriks, J. (1982). *Neurosci. Lett.* **34**, 283.
——, Mason, R., and Meijer, J. (1983). *Fed. Proc.* **42**, 2790.
Halberg, F. (1959). *Z. Vitamin-Hormon-Fermentforsch.* **10**, 225.
Halberg, F., Visscher, M.B., and Bittner J.J. (1954). *Am. J. Physiol.* **179**, 229.
Harrington, J.M. (1978). *Shift work and health. A critical review of the literature.* HMSO, London.
Hetzel, M.R. and Clark T.J.H. (1978). In *Chronopharmacology* (ed. A. Reinberg and F. Halberg), p.213. Pergamon Press, Oxford.
Inouye, S.T. and Kawamura, H. (1979). *Proc. Natl. Acad. Sci. USA* **76**, 5962.
Klein, K.E. and Wegmann, H-M. (1979). In *Sleep, wakefulness and circadian rhythm*, AGARD Lecture Series No. 105, Chapter 10. AGARD.
Lydic, R., Schoene, W.C., Czeisler, C.A., and Moore-Ede, M.C. (1980). *Sleep* **2**, 355.
Mills, J.N., Minors, D.S., and Waterhouse, J.M. (1974). *J. Physiol.* **240**, 567.
Mills, J.N., Minors, D.S., and Waterhouse, J.M. (1978*a*). *Chronobiologia* **5**, 14.
Mills, J.N., Minors, D.S., and Waterhouse, J.M. (1978*b*). *J. Physiol.* **285**, 455.
Minors, D.S. and Waterhouse, J.M. (1981). *Circadian rhythms and the human.* Wright PSG, Bristol.
Moore-Ede, M.C. (1983). *Fed. Proc.* **42**, 2802.
Moore-Ede, M.C., Sulzman, F.M., and Fuller, C.A. (1982). *The clocks that time us.* Harvard University Press, Cambridge, Massachusetts.
Moore, R.Y. (1979*a*). *Endocrine rhythms* (ed. D.T. Kreiger), p.63. Raven, New York.
Moore, R.Y. (1979*b*). In *Biological rhythms and their central mechanism* (ed. M. Suda, O. Hayaishi, and H. Nakagawa), p.343. Elsevier/North-Holland Biomedical, Amsterdam.
Moore, R.Y. (1983). *Fed. Proc.* **42**, 2783.
Moore, R.Y. and Eichler, V.B. (1972). *Brain Res.* **42**, 201.
Moore R.Y. and Lenn, N.J. (1972). *J. comp. Neurol.* **146**, 1.
Palmer, J.D. (1976). *An introduction to biological rhythms.* Academic Press, San Francisco.
Prevost, R.J., Smolensky, M.H., Reinberg, A., Raymer, W.J., and McGovern, J.P. (1980). In *Recent advances in the chronobiology of allergy and immunology* (ed. M.H. Smolensky, A. Reinberg, and J.P. McGovern), p.237. Pergamon Press, Oxford.
Raisman, G. and Brown-Grant, K. (1977). *Proc. R. Soc. London* **B198**, 297.
Reinberg, A., Gervais, P., Chaussade, M., Fraboulet, G., and Duburque, B. (1983). *J. Allergy clin. Immunol.* **71**, 425.
Reinberg, A., Guillet, P., Gervais, P., Ghata, J., Vignaud, D., and Abulker, C. (1977). *Chronobiologia* **4**, 295.
Reinberg, A. and Smolensky, M.H. (1982). *Clin. Pharmacokinet.* **7**, 401.
Reinberg, A., Smolensky, M., and Levi, F. (1981). *Biomedicine* **34**, 171.
Reindl, K., Falliers, C., and Halberg, F. (1969). *Rass Neurol. Veget.* **23**, 5.
Richter, C.P. (1967). *Res. publ. Ass. Res. nerv. ment. Dis.* **45**, 8.
Rusak, B. (1977). *J. comp. Physiol.* **118**, 145.
Rusak, B. and Groos, G. (1982). *Science* **215**, 1407.

Rusak, B. and Zucker, I. (1979). *Physiol. Rev.* **59**, 449.
Rutenfranz, J., Knauth, P., and Colquhoun, W.P. (1976). *Ergonomics* **19**, 331.
Schwartz, W.J., Davidsen, L.C., and Smith, C.B. (1980). *J. comp. Neurol.* **189**, 157.
Schwartz, W.J. and Gainer, H. (1977). *Science* **197**, 1089.
Smolensky, M.H. and Halberg, F. (1977). In *Chronobiology in allergy and immunology* (ed. J.P. McGovern, M.H. Smolensky, and A. Reinberg), p.117. Springfield, Illinois.
Smolensky, M., Halberg, F., and Sargent, F. (1972). In *Advances in climatic physiology* (ed. S. Ito, K. Ogata, and H. Yoshimura), p.281. Igaku Shoin, Tokyo.
Smolensky, M.H., Reinberg, A., and Queng, J.T. (1981). *Ann. Allerg.* **47**, 234.
Stephan, F.K. and Zucker, I. (1972). *Proc. Natl. Acad. Sci. USA* **69**, 1583.
Sulzman, F.M., Fuller, C.A., and Moore-Ede, M.C. (1977). *Comp. Biochem. Physiol.* **A58**, 63.
Weitzman, E.D., Czeisler, C.A., and Moore-Ede, M.C. (1979). In *Biological rhythms and their central mechanism* (ed. M. Suda, O. Hayaishi, and H. Nakagawa), p.199. Elsevier/North Holland Biomedical, Amsterdam.
Wever, R. (1970). *Pflugers Arch.* **321**, 133.
Wever, R. (1975). *Int. J. Chronobiol.* **3**, 19.
Wever, R.A. (1979). *The circadian system of man. Results of experiments under temporal isolation.* Springer-Verlag, Berlin.

Discussion

Professor D.C. Flenley

In the isolation studies you must put the light on or off at some time. Isn't there a clue to timing from that?

Dr D. Minors

No, there is self-selection of light on or off.

Dr D.E. Stableforth

Are the sites said to be the site of the clock in your rats and mice the same as those which control the pituitary?

Dr D. Minors

It seems to be different because in rhesus and squirrel monkeys, lesions of the suprachiasmatic nuclei do not lead to a loss of all circadian rhythmicity, although some variables seem to lose their rhythmicity. It is those variables controlled by the Y oscillator, which normally controls the sleep/wakefulness rhythm. The rhythms controlled by the anterior pituitary such as cortisol seem to be controlled by the X oscillator.

Airway function and reactivity at night

M.R. HETZEL

Whittington and University College Hospitals, London, UK.

Introduction

Nocturnal asthma has long been recognized and was well described by Willis (1679) and Floyer (1698). It is only in recent years, however, with the introduction of peak flow rate monitoring, both in hospital and at home, that the extent to which airways obstruction can increase at night has been recognized. This is usually recognized as a fall in peak expiratory flow rate (PEFR) on waking; the 'morning dip' (Turner-Warwick 1977). There is some evidence that nocturnal asthma is associated with an increased risk of death from asthma (Hetzel *et al.* 1977*a*; *Lancet* 1983) and this is very plausible when one appreciates the severity of the nocturnal fall in PEFR seen in some patients.

The possible aetiology of nocturnal asthma is considered in other sections of this book. In this section I will highlight some studies on the physiological changes seen at night in asthmatics and normal subjects and other types of airflow limitation, which have helped us better to understand the underlying circadian rhythms in airway calibre and bronchial reactivity. A knowledge of these rhythms should help the clinician treating patients with asthma to reach a more logical approach to management.

Physiological changes in nocturnal and early morning asthma

In a hospital study of PEFR patterns in asthma patients, it was found that there was an apparent increased risk of sudden death from asthma if the fall in PEFR on waking at 06.00 hours was repeatedly greater than 50 per cent of the highest daily reading (PEFR was measured four-hourly from 06.00 to 22.00 hours) (Hetzel *et al.* 1977*a*). We subsequently studied patients in hospital who consistently showed morning dips of >25 per cent more clearly to define the changes in pulmonary physiology that were occurring in these patients and to relate them to the patterns of lung function test results noted in acute asthma (Woolcock and Read 1966). In 16 patients lung function tests were performed in the laboratory immediately after waking at 06.00 hours, having discontinued bronchodilator drugs after 22.00 hours the previous night. They were then repeated after 200 mcg salbutamol aerosol and performed once more at 14.00 hours. Results were analysed in terms of percentages of predicted normal values to allow for differing age, sex, and height. Comparison of results at 06.00 with those at 14.00 showed that PEFR, forced expiratory volume in 1 second (FEV_1), and specific conductance (SGAW) had fallen by a mean 33, 30.7, and 47 per cent of predicted values respectively. Functional residual capacity (FRC) and residual volume (RV) had risen by 23 and 49 per cent, respectively. Total lung capacity (TLC) increased by 0.02–1.84 l. The volume of gas trapping, expressed as VA/TLC per cent (VA; alveolar volume determined by helium dilution technique during 10 seconds breathhold), increased; thus this ratio fell from 89.1 to 74.5 per cent. Mid-expiratory flow rates fell from 32.5 to 20.5 per cent. After aerosol salbutamol at 06.00 hours, many patients improved dramatically and achieved results compatible with those subsequently seen at 14.00 hours. In four, however, little response was seen. Arterial blood gas samples at 06.00 (before salbutamol) and 14.00 showed much less variation with no real change in pH and PCO_2. PO_2 fell a mean 0.57 kPa (4.3 mm Hg) at 06.00 and the alveolar-arterial oxygen tension gradient was persistently wide at 4.8 kPa (36 mm Hg) at 06.00 and 4.3 kPa (32.3 mm Hg) at 14.00 hours. Response in mid-expiratory flow rate to a mixture of 21 per cent oxygen in 79 per cent helium showed that two patients were helium responders (>20 per cent improvement (Despas et al. 1972)) at all times, seven were consistent non-responders, but seven had a variable response.

Thus changes in lung volumes and spirometry of an order compatible with an acute asthma attack (Woolcock and Read 1966) can occur every night in patients with nocturnal asthma and these patients may be completely asymptomatic with normal spirometry during the day. Although PEFR and FEV_1 may be normal at 14.00 hours, the persistence of a wide alveolar–arterial oxygen tension gradient, high RV, but near-normal SGAW seen at this time suggest residual small-airways obstruction. The rhythm in PEFR may therefore be attributable to changes in large airways with persistent small-airway obstruction throughout the 24 hours. The variable response to oxy-helium mixture in the flow-volume curve was unhelpful in defining the site of airflow limitation. The validity of this test is, however, questionable at the low flow rates generated by some of these patients in the early morning, since laminar flow tends to predominate at low flow rates even in larger airways.

This question has been considered again in a study in children (Mak et al. 1982) which concluded that circadian variation occurs equally in small and large airways. Eight children with asthma were studied at 08.00–09.00 hours and 17.00–18.00 hours on 10 consecutive days. Response to oxy-helium mixture was consistent at both times with a ratio of mid-expiratory flow rate ($V\dot{V}_{50}$) on He–O_2/air of mean value 1.29 in the morning and 1.31 in the afternoon. Three children were consistent non-responders and five were consistent responders. The authors found that the maximal expiratory flow curves increased proportionately at all lung volumes in the afternoon and concluded that airway calibre changed throughout the bronchial tree. It must be noted, however, that these children had less severe asthma than in the adult study, circadian variation in PEFR and FEV_1 was less marked, and no other lung function tests were carried out.

The observation of a dramatic response to aerosol salbutamol in the early morning, even in cases of severe nocturnal asthma, has been made in several studies (Hetzel et al. 1977b; Fairfax et al. 1980; Barnes et al. 1982) but much less effect is seen from oral or intravenous salbutamol; perhaps because the beta$_2$-receptors are more accessible by the aerosol route. In the minority who fail to respond to aerosol salbutamol (Hetzel et al. 1977b), this might be because mucus plugging prevents adequate aerosol penetration. Absence of mucus plugging might be the only pathological difference between a nocturnal asthma attack and a typical acute attack requiring hospital admission but it is possible that mucus plugging can develop rapidly. It is rare not to see mucus plugging at post mortem in deaths from asthma, even if they are sudden (Hetzel et al. 1977a; Speizer et al. 1968).

The normal circadian rhythm in airway calibre

Any hypothesis as to the cause of nocturnal asthma must take into account its similarity to the normal circadian rhythm in airway calibre. This was first detected in studies which involved accurate measurements in the respiratory laboratory over short periods of time. It is, however, quite easy to demonstrate this low-amplitude rhythm with a peak flow meter alone; provided a longitudinal study over several days, with an adequate spacing of readings, is used.

Table 1 summarises some of these earlier studies: many of which were transverse experiments lasting less than 24 hours. Lewinsohn *et al.* (1960) studied FEV_1 in normal and asthmatic subjects between 06.00 and 08.00 hours and compared an increase in FEV_1 of 2.9 per cent of the highest reading (at 08.00) in normals with 30–60 per cent in patients with airways obstruction. Guberan *et al.* (1969) studied FEV_1 in workers on different shifts on different days to construct an overall picture of their diurnal variation. Mc Dermott (1966) studied variations in inspira-

Table 1
Normal circadian variation in lung function tests

Test	Author	Amplitude	n	Acrophase
FEV_1	Lewinsohn *et al.* (1960)	2.9 per cent	5	08.00
	Guberan *et al.* (1969)	0.15 L	19	14.00
RAW	Mc Dermott (1966)	2.04 kPa L^{-1}s	9	08.00
	Gaultier *et al.* (1977)*	1.48 cm H$_2$O L^{-1}	14	03.30–05.30
SGAW	Kerr (1973)	0.83 s^{-1} kPa^{-1}	6	12.00
TLco	Cinkotai and Thomson (1966)	−1.2 to −2.2 per cent/hr	24	08.00
PEFR	Reindle *et al.* (1970)	24 L min^{-1}	1	17.00
	Reinberg *et al.* (1970)	20–70 per cent	3	10.00–16.00
Dynamic Compliance	Gaultier *et al.* (1977)*	dyn m^{-1}cm H$_2$O^{-1}	14	09.31

Amplitude is shown in raw values or as percentages of mean value. Acrophase is best possible estimate of time of peak value in rhythm, but must be approximate only in studies lasting less than 24 hours. *Studies carried out in chidren.

tory resistance in nine normals and found it was highest at 08.00. Cinkotai and Thomson (1966) demonstrated that gas transfer factor for carbon monoxide falls during the day and this cannot be explained by a change from the sleeping to erect posture. Longer studies are needed to accurately quantify the rhythm in airway calibre and identify its phase. Kerr (1973), though principally interested in effects of air pollution, provided elegant data on airways resistance and lung volumes in six subjects over a six-day period in environmentally controlled chambers. This study demonstrated an amplitude of 0.083 cm H$_2$O^{-1} (0.83 s^{-1}kPa^{-1}) in specific conductance, 0.305 L in FRC, 0.17 L in TLC, and 0.2 L in RV.

PEFR, although a less accurate measurement, is ideal for study of the rhythm in airway calibre in normals because the portable peak flow meter can be used at home over long periods of time to make up for its relatively low accuracy. Reindl *et al.* (1970) and Reinberg *et al.* (1970) used PEFR in normal subjects and found highest readings in the early afternoon.

We subsequently studied a larger group of normal subjects (Hetzel and Clark 1980) in order to better define the amplitude and phase of the normal circadian rhythm in airway calibre. 221 normal subjects were recruited whose ages ranged from 10 to 84 years. There were 107 males and 114 females. On questionnaires they had no history of cardiorespiratory disease, were on no medication other than the oral contraceptive, and could achieve a PEFR within two standard deviations of predicted normal values. Three attempts at PEFR with a Wright peak flow gauge were recorded on waking, leaving for work, coming home from work, and at bedtime for seven consecutive days. Cosinor analysis (Halberg *et al.* 1964) was used to analyse the raw data for rhythmicity. This uses a multiple regression programme to regress PEFR on time and test the goodness of fit of a sinusoidal waveform with a period of around 24 hours to the raw data. The programme quotes the statistical significance of rhythmicity in the raw data, the amplitude of the rhythm and its phase, quoted as the acrophase or time of the highest value in the 24-hour cycle.

145 subjects (65.6 per cent) had a significant PEFR rhythm. Their mean amplitude was 8.3 per cent of each individual's average daily PEFR (standard deviation ±5.2 per cent). There was a clear pattern of distribution of the timing of the acrophase with most subjects showing an acrophase between 14.00 and 18.00 hours (mean acrophase 15.57 hours). In the remaining 76 normal subjects, whose data did not reveal rhythmicity at a statiscitally significant level, the distribution of estimated phase of their rhythms was, nevertheless, very similar to that seen in the other subjects with significant rhythms. This suggests that all normal subjects probably have a rhythm in PEFR but in these 76 subjects its amplitude was too low for totally effective detection on the frequency of readings employed. Clearly, no pattern of distribution of phase would be expected if no true rhythm was being detected in these subjects.

Fifteen subjects were also available for study with flow-volume loops at 09.30, 12.00, and 17.30 hours for five consecutive days in the respiratory laboratory. Eleven had previously shown significant rhythms in PEFR at home. No single measurement from the flow-volume loop showed rhythmicity in as many of them, but in the four subjects who had not had significant rhythms at home, significant rhythms were now detectable in some components of the loop. This further supports the view that all normals have a rhythm in airway calibre, but also illustrates that the simple measurement of PEFR over a wider 'window' of the period of wakefulness at home is more valuable than more complex tests in the laboratory which cannot so easily be performed throughout the waking day.

A similar protocol of PEFR measurements was carried out in 56 asthma patients; either in hospital or immediately after discharge home. All had wheezy breathlessness, and a >20 per cent improvement in PEFR or FEV_1 after bronchodilator drugs or a >50 per cent improvement in PEFR during their hospital admission. All showed significant rhythmicity on cosinor analysis with a mean amplitude of 50.9 per cent (±S.D. 41.7 per cent). Mean acrophase was at 15.57 hours and the distribution of phase was very similar to that seen in the normal subjects.

There was no convincing relationship in the normal subjects in this study between amplitude of the PEFR rhythm and age, smoking history, history of atopy, family history of asthma, or sex; although the subjects over the age of 70 years did have a significantly higher amplitude than all other age groups.

These results suggest that nocturnal asthma represents an amplification of a normal circadian rhythm in airway calibre since the two rhythms only differ in amplitude. Amplitude apparently relates to the degree of bronchial lability in the asthma patient. On these results, normal subjects would not be expected to have an amplitude of >20 per cent (mean value ±2SD; 8.3±10.4 per cent). This might be a useful criterion for making a diagnosis of asthma on PEFR monitoring alone. A number of other studies now need to be considered in relation to the question of what order of PEFR amplitude is indicative of asthma.

Dawkins and Muers (1981) used similar methods to evaluate the effects of smoking and chronic bronchitis on the PEFR rhythm. Some previous studies (Zedda and Sartorelli 1971; Connolly 1979) had included analysis of PEFR diurnal variation in cases labelled as chronic bronchitis but the possibility of an asthmatic component in these patients was not fully excluded. Dawkins and Muers selected smokers with no past or family history of asthma, rhinitis, conjunctivitis, or atopy and with no history of wheeze on exposure to allergens, exercise, or cold air. Skin prick tests were negative, IgE levels normal, and they had no sputum eosinophilia. Twelve patients satisfying these criteria recorded PEFR at 07.00, 08.00, 12.00, 18.00, and 23.00 hours for 14 days. The bronchodilator response to 40 mcg ipratropium bromide and 200 mcg salbutamol was measured at the beginning and end of the study. Cosinor analysis showed a significant rhythm in PEFR in 10 patients with a mean amplitude of 8.6 per cent of individual average daily PEFR (± SD 5.7 per cent). Thus the amplitude of the PEFR rhythm in patients with irreversible airflow limitation from chronic bronchitis and emphysema was very similar to that of normal subjects (Hetzel and Clark 1980) which further strengthens the view that the labile airways of the asthmatic account for his greater amplitude. A further important point in this study was that the response to salbutamol and ipratropium was smaller than the natural diurnal variation in PEFR; thus one should beware of inadvertently attributing this variation to a true benefit from bronchodilator therapy in chronic airflow limitation.

Johnston *et al.* (1983) used cosinor analysis to study PEFR amplitude in asthmatic children. From a survey of Croydon schoolchildren in which a postal questionnaire was sent to parents of 5096 children, replies were received from 4447 (87 per cent) and 495 of these (11 per cent) reported wheezing or asthma in the last 12 months. 284 wheezy children were selected for home interview. 102 of them had been wheezy within the last month and were asked to keep a diary card of symptoms. 64 of 85 children who successfully kept diary cards then agreed to a second period of symptom monitoring, together with PEFR measurement at 08.00, 16.00, and 21.00 hours for 12 days.

Nocturnal asthma appeared to be much less common than in adult studies (Hetzel and Clark 1980). Only 14 of the 64 children had a significant rhythm on cosinor analysis and their mean amplitude was 20 per cent. In the whole group the mean amplitude was 12 per cent (range 1.1–52.8 per cent). As in the adult studies, the distribution of phase was similar to normals, adult asthmatics, and chronic bronchitics with the majority showing an acrophase between 12.00 and 17.00 hours. Many asthmatic children that one sees in hospital out-patient wards appear to frequently complain of wheeze or cough at night and one suspects that there may be no true difference between the amplitudes of child and adult asthmatics but that the difference results from Johnston *et al.* (1983) having attempted a proper community survey whereas the adult studies cited are from highly selected groups of hospital patients. Nevertheless, these children had significant symptoms. 87 per cent had missed some school in the last year and 31 per cent had missed more than six weeks. 80 per cent had attended their GP for wheezing in the last year and 57 per cent were on therapy during the study. A further factor may be the 'window' through which the PEFR data was obtained. This was 13/24 hours (08.00–21.00) compared with 16–18 hours of the 24-hour cycle in the adult studies (Hetzel and Clark 1980; Dawkins and Muers 1981); thus the shorter period of wakefulness in children could have led to some underestimation of amplitude.

It is not, therefore, possible to define the threshold amplitude for a diagnosis of asthma at present. The problem is increased by the different methods of analysis, timing of measurements, duration of study, and criteria of selection of patients used by different workers. Cosinor analysis is the most reliable means of ensuring that a true rhythm is distinguished from biological noise, but the PEFR variation is often measured directly as a percentage of the highest daily value or of the mean daily value. This tends to overestimate the amplitude of the rhythm, although the two different methods of analysis are reasonably compatible except when amplitude is very large. For example, quoting amplitude from direct reading of raw data using the morning fall in PEFR as a percentage of the highest daily reading, Connolly (1979) found a mean amplitude of 29 per cent in asthmatics in hospital and Ryan *et al.* (1982) quote 7.6 per cent in out-patient asthmatics. Amplitude thus varies widely in asthmatics and, if they are in remission, their amplitude may fall within the normal range. On the basis of a reasonably-sized study in normals (Hetzel and Clark 1980), however, it seems unlikely that an amplitude of >20 per cent is normal, but a lower amplitude may be seen in normals or asymptomatic asthmatics.

Circadian variation in airway reactivity

De Vries *et al.* (1962) considered that variations in bronchial reactivity might underlie the clinical phenomenon of nocturnal asthma. They studied 11 young asthmatics with positive skin tests to common allergens and reversible airways obstruction and five older patients with more severe and chronic airways obstruction whom they described as chronic asthmatic bronchitis and emphysema, who had marked reduction in FEV_1 and VC and a RV/TLC per cent ratio of >40 per cent. Increasing concentrations of nebulised histamine were given up to a maximum dose of 32 mg/ml, until the threshold concentration to cause a >10 per cent fall in FEV_1 was determined. This threshold concentration was measured at 12.00, 16.00, 20.00, 24.00, 04.00, 08.00, and 12.00 hours. In both groups of patients a significant fall in the threshold for histamine response was found between 20.00 and 04.00 hours with a median threshold of 1 mg ml^{-1} in the young asthmatics and 0.5 mg ml^{-1} in the older patients. During the day, thresholds rose to 4–8 mg ml^{-1} in both groups. Thus there was little apparent difference in bronchial reactivity between these two groups of patients. Circadian variation in baseline values for FEV_1 was relatively small so that the changes in histamine threshold were unlikely to be an artefact from the degree of airways obstruction already prevailing at the time of challenge. In the young asthmatics FEV_1 rose from 1.67 L at 04.00 to 2.14 L at 12.00 hours; compared with 0.76 L and 0.9 L, respectively, in the older patients. Thus a nocturnal rise in bronchial reactivity coincides with the rise in airways resistance at night and undoubtedly contributes to it as patients become more sensitive to any allergic or physical factors to which they might be exposed at night. Since nocturnal asthma is common in intrinsic asthma (Clark and Hetzel 1977) and the PEFR rhythm persists, although with a lower amplitude, in atopic asthmatics in allergen-free environments (Reinberg *et al.* 1970), it is unlikely, however, that the rhythm in bronchial reactivity could be the sole cause of nocturnal asthma.

Similar results are seen with other forms of bronchial challenge. Reinberg *et al.* (1974) compared the threshold dose of acetylcholine to produce a fall in FEV_1 of >15 per cent in eight normal subjects and six asthmatics at 08.00, 15.00, 19.00, and 23.00 hours. These times were studied on separate days and in random order. Cosinor analysis showed a mean FEV_1 of 3.35 L with an amplitude of 7.4 per cent and an acrophase of 15.59 hours in the normal subjects; compared with results of 2.23 L, 10 per cent and 15.56 hours, respectively, in the asthmatics. The mean threshold dose of acetylcholine was 6460 mcg, with an amplitude of 60 per cent of the mean value and an acrophase at 14.54 hours in the normals, compared with 398 mcg, 40 per cent and 13.36 hours, respectively, in the asthmatics. Thus as for histamine challenge, greatest bronchial reactivity to acetylcholine is seen at night, but it is also notable that, although the asthmatics had a lower threshold for acetylcholine, the amplitude of the rhythm in bronchial reactivity to acetylcholine was no greater in asthmatics than normals.

Gervais *et al.* (1977) also demonstrated a rhythm in bronchial reactivity to inhaled allergens in sensitized asthmatics. Four patients with asthma provoked by house dust were studied in rooms with filtration systems to reduce background allergen exposure. Over a 10-day study period they were challenged every other day to determine the threshold dose of house dust extract to produce a >20 per cent fall in FEV_1 15 minutes after challenge at 08.00, 15.00, 19.00, and 23.00 hours; one time only being studied on each study day. Bronchial reactivity was greatest at 23.00 hours, when bronchoconstriction was also most persistent, and least at 15.00 hours.

The relationship between bronchial reactivity and the amplitude of variation in PEFR has been further clarified by Ryan *et al.* (1982). They studied nine normal subjects, five patients with a past history of asthma, and 27 patients with current asthma symptoms. Bronchial hyperreactivity to histamine was measured as PC_{20}; the concentration of inhaled histamine needed to cause a >20 per cent fall in FEV_1. The amplitude of the rhythm in PEFR was determined by home monitoring and the response to salbutamol by inhalation in the morning was measured.

Bronchial reactivity was much greater in the asthmatics, with a mean PC_{20} of 0.87 mg ml^{-1}, than in the asymptomatic asthmatics (25.6 mg ml^{-1}) and normal subjects (45 mg ml^{-1}). There was a significant correlation between PC_{20} and PEFR in the early morning, so that the lower the PC_{20} (more reactive airways) the lower the morning PEFR (greater amplitude in circadian rhythm) with a correlation coefficient $r = 0.82$. Moreover, there was also an inverse correlation between PC_{20} and the improvement in morning PEFR after salbutamol (i.e. the greater the bronchial reactivity, the greater the response to bronchodilator drugs). The amplitude of diurnal variation in PEFR, measured as a percentage of the highest daily reading, also showed an inverse correlation with PC_{20} ($r = -0.75$ and $r = -0.81$, respectively).

Thus, if one accepts response to bronchodilator drugs and PC_{20} as indices of bronchial lability, these results support the hypothesis that nocturnal asthma represents amplification of a normal circadian rhythm in airway calibre by the asthmatic's labile airways, and the amplitude of variation of PEFR and the fall in PEFR in the early morning, can be used as objective measures of bronchial lability and the standard of control of the patient's asthma. The problem with this study is, of course, the difference in the baseline levels of PEFR between normals and asthmatics on which the PC_{20} response is based. This study also showed a rather low amplitude in the PEFR rhythm of the asthmatic subjects; mean amplitudes were 8.0 per cent of highest daily reading in the asymptomatic asthmatics, 21.9 per cent in symptomatic asthmatics, and 6.7 per cent in the normals subjects. As discussed earlier, this outpatient study suggests that asthmatics who are clinically well controlled may have no greater diurnal variation in PEFR than normal subjects.

These observations might explain the common observation in recovery from an acute asthma attack in hospital that, initially, when PEFR is low, there is little diurnal variation in PEFR. Subsequently, as PEFR starts to increase with response to treatment, the amplitude of PEFR increases and may become large with symptoms of nocturnal wheezing. Finally, with full recovery from the attack and a PEFR which represents the patient's usual best results, the amplitude of diurnal variation may be much smaller again. It would seem that bronchial lability is temporarily increased as patients recover from acute asthma and at this stage considerable amplification of the underlying circadian rhythm occurs and manifests itself as morning dips in the PEFR chart. During this period of increased bronchial lability, sudden death is more likely than at other times (Hetzel *et al.* 1977*a*).

Conclusions

There are normal circadian rhythms in airway calibre and in the reactivity of the airways. These have a similar phase so that, at night or in the early morning, resting airway calibre is reduced and bronchial reactivity is increased. Superimposed on these normal rhythms, the more labile airways of the asthmatic cause the phenomena of nocturnal asthma and 'morning dips' and the severity of these can be considered as indicators of good or poor control of asthma. While the amplitude of the PEFR rhythm is different in asthma and normal subjects, there is no other clear difference between the rhythms in airway calibre and reactivity in normals, chronic bronchitis, and emphysema and asthma; nor is there any difference in relation to children versus adults.

The concept of nocturnal asthma as a state of increased bronchial lability has important implications for treatment. While it may at first seem logical to give treatment at night, treatment on a regular basis during the waking day might be expected to reduce bronchial lability and indirectly control nocturnal symptoms. In the author's experience this concept does seem to be an effective way of treating at least the milder cases of nocturnal asthma.

References

Barnes, P.J., Greening, A.P., Neville, L., Timmers, J., and Poole, G. (1982). *Lancet* **i**, 299.
Cinkotai, F.F. and Thomson, M.L. (1966). *J. appl. Physiol.* **21**, 539.
Clark, T.J.H. and Hetzel, M.R. (1977). *Br. J. Dis. Chest* **71**, 87.
Connolly, C.K. (1979). *Br. J. Dis. Chest.* **73**, 357.
Dawkins, K.D. and Muers, M.F. (1981). *Thorax* **36**, 618.
Despas, P.J., Leroux, M., and Macklem, P.T. (1972). *J. clin. Invest.* **51**, 3235.
De Vries, K., Goei, J.T., Booy-Noord, H., and Orie, N.G.M. (1962). *Int. Arch. Allergy* **20**, 93.
Fairfax, A.J., Mc Nabb, W.R., Davies, H.J., and Spiro, S.G. (1980). *Thorax* **35**, 526.
Floyer, J. (1698). *A treatise of the asthma.* Wilkin & Innys, London.
Gaultier, C., Reinberg, A., and Girard, F. (1977). *Resp. Physiol.* **31**, 169.
Gervais, P., Reinberg, A., Gervais, C., Smolensky, M., and De France, O. (1977). *J. Allergy clin. Immunol.* **59**, 207.
Guberan, E., Williams, M.K., Walford, J., and Smith, M.M. (1969). *Br. J. indust. Med.* **26**, 121.
Halberg, F., Diffley, M., Stein, M., Panofsky, H., and Adkins, G. (1964). *Ann. NY Acad. Sci.* **115**, 695.
Hetzel, M.R. and Clark, T.J.H. (1980). *Thorax* **35**, 732.
Hetzel, M.R., Clark, T.J.H., and Branthwaite, M.A. (1977). *Br. med. J.* **i**, 808.
Hetzel, M.R., Clark, T.J.H., and Houston, K. (1977). *Thorax* **32**, 418.
Johnston, I.D.A., Anderson, H.R., and Patel, S. (1983). *Thorax* **38**, 230.
Kerr, H.D. (1973). *Arch. environ. Hlth* **26**, 144.
Lancet (1983). Editorial. *Lancet* **i**, 220.
Lewinsohn, H.C., Capel, L.H., and Smart, J. (1960). *Br. med. J.* **1**, 462.
Mak, H. *et al.* (1982). *Br. J. Dis. Chest* **76**, 51.
Mc Dermott, M. (1966). *J. Physiol.* **186**, 90P.
Reinberg, A. *et al.* (1970). *La Presse Médicale* **78**, 1817.
Reinberg, A., Gervais, P., Morin, M., and Abulker, C. (1974). In *Chronobiology* (ed. L.E. Scheving, F. Halberg, and J.E. Pauly), p.174. Igaku Shoin, Tokyo.
Reindl, K., Falliers, C., Halberg, F., Chai, H., Hillman, D., and Nelson, W. (1970). *Rass. Neurol. Vegetat.* **23**, 5.
Ryan, G., Latimer, K.M., Dolovich, J., and Hargreaves, F.E. (1982). *Thorax* **37**, 423.
Speizer, F.E., Doll, R., and Heaf, P. (1968). *Br. med. J.* **1**, 335.
Turner-Warwick, M. (1977). *Br. J. Dis. Chest* **71**, 73.
Willis, T. (1679). *Pharmacutiae rationalis.* Dring, Harper, & Leigh, London.
Woolcock, A.J. and Read, J. (1966). *Am. J. Med.* **41**, 259.
Zedda, S. and Sartorelli, E. (1971). *Respiration* **28**, 158.

Discussion

Professor D.C. Flenley

A lot of your work is based upon four measurements and you then impose a sinusoidal pattern. If something happened at 4 a.m. which was outside the time you saw your pattern you would miss it entirely because you make no direct measurements then.

Dr M. Hetzel

It is not a very satisfactory model because if you take frequent points of measurement the sinusoidal shape is only an approximation. Asthmatics seem to plunge down quite quickly, but if you could devise a better mathematical model we would use it. In the epidemiological study of children quoted, one of the reasons that the amplitude appears to be lower may be that the window through which you are looking, during which children are awake, is much shorter than that in adults. That would automatically reduce the effect of amplitude.

Dr G. Laszlo

You said that during nocturnal dips or morning dips asthmatics are as bad as when they are brought into hospital with acute severe asthma. Full lung function results during this sort of dip show that the vital capacity falls from 100 to 75 per cent, which is not what happens in acute severe asthma. The difference between having morning asthma and having acute severe asthma is that vital capacity correlates with blood gases and the peak flow doesn't in this situation.

Dr M. Hetzel

The important point is simply the severity of the change that does occur. The vital capacity certainly does drop quite dramatically in these patients and, although the mean changes in blood gases were small, some individuals were very hypoxic at 6 a.m. with PO_2 values of 50 mm Hg. Some of those patients were unaware of how severe their asthma was at that time.

Dr I.S. Petheram

I wonder if in your large study of 220 patients you saw any who had the exact opposite of the phase you describe clearly?

Dr M. Hetzel

I have come across one or two patients who show 'evening dipping', the peak flow being lowest in the evening and highest on waking.

Autonomic control of the airways and nocturnal asthma

P.J. BARNES

Department of Medicine (Respiratory Division), Royal Postgraduate Medical School, Hammersmith Hospital, London W12 OHS, UK

Although wheezing at night and in the early morning has been a recognized feature of asthma since the earliest descriptions of the disease, it is only recently that the underlying mechanisms have been clarified. There is now considerable evidence that nocturnal asthma represents an exaggeration of the normal diurnal variation in airway calibre (Hetzel 1981; Barnes 1984). Amplification of the normal rhythm is related to hyperreactivity of the airways in asthma and there is a close relationship between the amplitude of 'morning dipping' and bronchial reactivity to inhaled histamine (Ryan *et al.* 1982). Nocturnal wheezing may therefore be regarded as a manifestation of bronchial hyperreactivity. Moreover the bronchoconstrictor response to inhaled histamine (De Vries *et al.* 1962) and acetylcholine (Reinberg and Gervais 1972) is greater in the early morning than during the day. This implies that the underlying mechanism of nocturnal asthma is likely to be that which determines the change in calibre of normal airways, and that the marked diurnal change in bronchomotor tone is the result of bronchial hyperreactivity in asthma (Fig. 1).

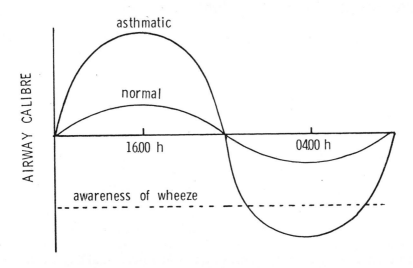

Fig. 1. *Nocturnal asthma represnts an exaggeration of the diurnal variation in airway calibre.*

Autonomic control of the airways

Airway tone is regulated by the autonomic nervous system (Nadel and Barnes 1984), and it is therefore possible that autonomic nervous mechanisms may be responsible for diurnal changes in bronchomotor tone. This speculation is not new and the seventeenth century physician John Floyer, himself an asthmatic, believed that wheezing occured at night 'when nerves are filled with windy spirits'. Because asthmatics show exaggerated constrictor responses to a wide variety of stimuli, there has been speculation that autonomic control of the airway is abnormal in asthma, with enhancement of excitatory pathways or diminution of inhibitory mechanisms (*Lancet* 1982). Human airways are densely innervated by cholinergic nerves, which are carried in the vagus nerve and synapse in ganglia within the airway wall (Richardson 1979). Activation of cholinergic nerves produces bronchoconstriction, which is inhibited by the cholinergic antagonist atropine. By contrast, the sympathetic nerve supply to human airways is very sparse, with no direct innervation of airway smooth muscle (Richardson 1979). However ß-adrenoceptor agonists potently relax human-airway smooth muscle *in vitro* (Barnes *et al*. 1984), and these ß-receptors must therefore be regulated by circulating catecholamines (Barnes 1983). In addition to a direct effect on airway smooth muscle, ß-agonists also inhibit allergen-induced release of mediators from human lung fragments (Butchers *et al*. 1980) and isolated mast cells (Peters *et al*. 1982) in vitro. In animals ß-agonists also inhibit neurotransmission through cholinergic ganglia and nerves (Skoogh 1983; Vermeire and Vanhoutte 1979), and may therefore produce bronchodilatation indirectly by modulating cholinergic tone. ß-adrenoceptor agonists may cause bronchoconstriction in asthmatic, but not in normal subjects, suggesting that ß-adrenergic contractile responses may be increased in asthma (Snashall *et al*. 1978; Black *et al*. 1982). A third nervous system, which is neither adrenergic nor cholinergic, relaxes human-airway smooth muscle *in vitro*, but the functional significance of this nervous system, or whether it is abnormal in asthma has not yet been determined (Richardson 1981).

ß-adrenoceptor function at night

Because ß-agonists reverse asthmatic bronchoconstriction it was logical to suggest that there might be a defect in ß-receptor function in asthma (Sventivanyi 1968). There is no convincing evidence for a significant primary abnormality in ß-receptor function in asthma however, although it remains uncertain whether secondary impairment in ß-adrenergic responsiveness may occur as a result of asthma (*Lancet* 1982; Barnes *et al*. 1984). A possible explanation of nocturnal asthma may be that ß-receptor function is impaired at night and the observation that ß-agonists are not very effective in treating nocturnal asthma tends to support this contention (Fairfax *et al*. 1980). To test this proposition ß-adrenergic responsiveness was measured at different times during a 24-hour period in a group of asthmatics who complained of nocturnal wheeze. No difference was found in heart rate, blood pressure, or plasma cyclic AMP response to graded infusions of adrenaline at different times (Barnes *et al*. 1982). The bronchodilator responses to both infused and inhaled adrenaline were greater at the time of maximal bronchoconstriction at 04.00 h because the baseline peak flow value was lower. These results therefore suggest that there is no significant diurnal change in ß-adrenergic responsiveness in asthma, and that ß-receptor dysfunction at night is not the underlying mechanism of nocturnal asthma. However a reduced density of ß-receptors on circulating lymphocytes has been found in the been found in the early morning compared with during the evening (Titinchi *et al.* 1984), but measurement of ß-receptors on circulating blood cells may have little relevance to asthmatic airways.

Circulating adrenaline

In the absence of direct sympathetic innervation, human-airway smooth muscle ß-receptors must be regulated physiologically by circulating catecholamines (Barnes 1981, 1983). Noradrenaline in plasma is derived from overspill of sympathetic nerve activity and has no significant physiological effect in man, whereas adrenaline secreted by the adrenal medulla has potent effects on $ß_2$-receptors (FitzGerald *et al.* 1980). Although resting concentrations of adrenaline are not elevated in asthmatic patients (Barnes *et al.* 1982), the fact that asthmatics develop bronchoconstriction with ß-adrenoceptor antagonists suggests that circulating adrenaline protects against bronchoconstriction (Barnes *et al.* 1984).

There is a circadian variation in catecholamine excretion, with lowest amounts excreted at night (Townshend and Smith 1973), and in asthmatic subjects the time of maximal bronchoconstriction coincides with the period when urinary excretion of catecholamines is lowest (Soutar *et al.* 1977). Measurements of plasma adrenaline have confirmed this association, with the lowest concentrations of adrenaline at 04.00 h, corresponding to the time of maximal bronchoconstriction (Barnes *et al.* 1980). Plasma cyclic AMP concentration, which probably reflects generalised ß-receptor stimulation by adrenaline (FitzGerald *et al.* 1980), follows a similar pattern. The fall in plasma adrenaline in normal subjects, studied under the same conditions, is identical. This means that the same fall in endogenous adrenaline is associated with bronchoconstriction in asthmatic subjects but not in normal subjects. This is analogous to the effect of ß-blockers, which inhibit endogenous adrenaline, and cause bronchospasm in asthmatic subjects, but have no effect on airway function in normal subjects (Barnes *et al.* 1984).

Adrenaline is secreted from the adrenal medulla and rapidly cleared from the plasma (FitzGerald *et al.* 1980). As no change in plasma clearance of adrenaline has been found at different times during a 24-hour period, the fall in plasma adrenaline at night must be due to reduced secretion from the adrenal gland (Fig. 2). Secretion of adrenaline is regulated by the hypothalamus (Ungar and Phillips 1983), an area implicated in the control of several circadian rhythms which seems to be the central clock (Moore-Ede *et al.* 1983).

The fall in circulating adrenaline at night may produce bronchoconstriction by a reduction in endogenous stimulation of $ß_2$-receptors on airway smooth muscle, or indirectly by effects on other cells in the airway. ß-agonists inhibit mediator secretion from human lung mast cells, and it is therefore possible that withdrawal of endogenous ß-agonist stimulation by adrenaline may be associated with an increased release of bronchoconstrictor mediators from airway mast cells. In support of this a rise in plasma histamine concentration is found in asthmatic subjects at the time of maximal bronchoconstriction at 04.00 h, and a close correlation between the rise in plasma histamine and the fall in plasma adrenaline and peak flow (Barnes *et al.* 1980). No such rise in plasma histamine concentration is found in normal subjects at night, and the increase in asthmatics may represent the propensity of 'sensitized' mast cells in asthmatics to more readily release mediators. Histamine has been used as an index of mediator release, but presumably other constrictor mediators, such as leucotrienes and prostaglandin D_2, and chemotactic factors would also be secreted.

Although the coincidence of circadian rhythms does not mean that they are causally related, some evidence that the rise in plasma histamine is related to the fall in endogenous adrenaline is provided by the demonstration that when adrenaline is infused in a low concentration (0.01 µg/kg/min) at 04.00 h to compensate for the fall

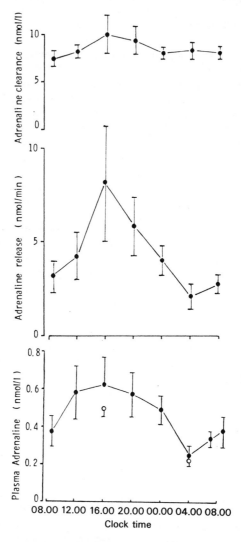

Fig. 2. *Circadian variations in endogenous plasma adrenaline (bottom panel), adrenaline release (middle panel), and adrenaline clearance (top panel) in five asthmatic subjects (mean ±SEM). Values of plasma adrenaline in five normal subjects are also shown (open circles) in the bottom panel.*

in endogenous adrenaline concentration, there is a fall in plasma histamine and an increase in peak flow (Barnes *et al.* 1980). Interpretation of plasma histamine measurements must be made with some caution however, as it is likely that they reflect release from circulating basophils, rather than from airway mast cells (Ind *et al.* 1983), and the assumption is that these cells behave in the same way.

ß-agonists have an inhibitory effect on cholinergic neurotransmission in animals, both at the level of cholinergic ganglia in the airway wall (Skoogh 1983) and on postganglionic pathways (Vermeire and Vanhoutte). Thus a fall in endogenous adrenaline may release a braking effect on cholinergic bronchoconstrictor tone and the effect of this would be magnified if there were evidence, as in asthma, of hyperactivity of cholinergic pathways. Indirect support for this is provided by the demonstration that bronchoconstriction produced by ß-blockers in asthma is abolished by anticholinergic drugs (Grieco and Pierson 1971).

Steroids and autonomic control

It was suggested several years ago that the circadian rhythm in endogenous corticosteroids may underly nocturnal asthma (Reinberg *et al.* 1963), but there is no direct relationship between the time of fall in plasma cortisol and increased bronchoconstriction (Barnes *et al.* 1980; Soutar *et al.* 1975). Moreover an infusion of hydrocortisone, sufficient to abolish the circadian fall in plasma cortisol, fails to prevent nocturnal wheeze (Soutar *et al.* 1975). Although the lowest concentration of plasma cortisol is found at midnight and therefore precedes the lowest peak flow by four hours, both the onset and decay of steroid effects are delayed, so it is possible that endogenous steroid withdrawal may play a permissive role in nocturnal asthma. This could result from withdrawal of its anti-inflammatory effect on the airways, although this seems unlikely. Steroids increase the expression of pulmonary ß-receptors (Barnes *et al.* 1984), and a fall in cortisol concentration at night could therefore lead to a reduction in airway ß-receptor function. However, as discussed above, there is no evidence that ß-adrenergic function is reduced at night (Barnes *et al.* 1982). A third possibility is that steroids may influence the synthesis and secretion of adrenaline by the adrenal medulla, since in animals hypophysectomy, with the resultant fall in ACTH, leads to reduced adrenaline synthesis, as cortisol produced in the adrenal cortex is necessary for the function of the enzyme phenylethanolamine N-methyl transferase which converts noradrenaline to adrenaline in chromaffin cells of the adrenal medulla (Porohecky *et al.* 1971).

Cholinergic mechanisms

Blockade of cholinergic receptors by anticholinergic drugs such as atropine results in bronchodilatation in normal and asthmatic subjects, indicating a degree of resting cholinergic tone in human airways (Nadel and Barnes 1984). There is evidence that cholinergic bronchoconstriction is enhanced in asthma as the exaggerated bronchoconstrictor responses to inhaled challenges such as sulphur dioxide, cold air, and inert dusts are inhibited by cholinergic blockade. It is possible that changes in cholinergic tone may underly the diurnal variation in airway tone of normal and asthmatic subjects, and this would explain why the bronchoconstrictor response in asthmatics is exaggerated.

Such a circadian variation in cholinergic tone might be secondary to changes in plasma adrenaline, with the fall in endogenous ß-receptor stimulation at night leading to increased cholinergic bronchoconstriction. There could also be a reduction in central parasympathetic drive. A further possibility is that cholinergic pathways are activated at night by reflex mechanisms, such as stimulation of irritant receptors by inflammatory mediators like histamine, or by cooling (Chen and Chai 1982), or in some cases by reflux of gastric acid stimulating afferent-nerve fibres in the oesophagus (Goodall *et al.* 1981). There is no direct evidence for a circadian variation in cholinergic regulation of the airways, but some evidence that vagal tone to the heart, as judged by the sinus arrythmia gap, is increased at night. (Clarke *et al.* 1976). Furthermore there is a close relationship between a fall in heart rate during the night and the fall in peak expiratory flow (Barnes *et al.* 1982), indicating that increased vagal tone to the airways is a strong possibility. There is also preliminary evidence that anticholinergic drugs such as ipratropium bromide, given in large doses at night, may prevent nocturnal wheezing (Svedmyr N, personal communication).

Conclusions

There is now compelling evidence that nocturnal asthma may be explained by the coincidence of several circadian rhythms which interact in the airways. The fall in endogenous plasma adrenaline, the delayed effects of cortisol withdrawal, and an increase in cholinergic tone may all lead to bronchoconstriction at night and in the early morning (Fig. 3). In normal subjects this results in only small changes in airway

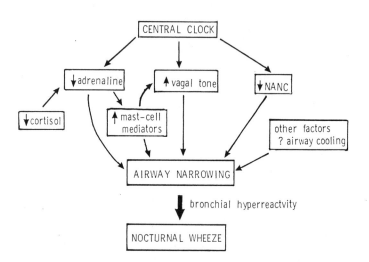

Fig. 3. Mechanisms of nocturnal asthma.

calibre, but in asthmatic patients these same changes produce pronounced bronchoconstriction, because of bronchial hyperreactivity. These changes may also be amplified in asthmatics by increased mediator release from sensitized airway mast cells.

Because there are several underlying mechanisms of nocturnal asthma, it is not surprising that treatment with a single drug may not be satisfactory and a combination of drugs is probably a more logical approach for the treatment of this troublesome symptom of asthma.

References

Barnes, P.J. (1981). *Clin. Physiol.* **1**, 89.
Barnes, P.J. (1983). *Eur. J. resp. Dis.* **64**, 559.
Barnes, P.J. (1984). *Br. med. J.* (in press).
Barnes, P., FitzGerald, G., Brown, M., and Dollery, C.T. (1980). *N. Engl. J. Med.* **303**, 263.
Barnes, P.J., FitzGerald, G.A., and Dollery, C.T. (1982). *Clin. Sci.* **62**, 349.
Barnes, P.J., Ind, P.W., and Brown, M.J. (1982). *Clin. Sci.* **62**, 661.
Barnes, P.J., Ind, P.W., and Dollery, C.T. (1984). In *Asthma: physiology, immunopharmacology and treatment* (ed. A.B. Kay, K.F. Austen and L.M. Lichtenstein), Academic Press, London and New York.
Black, J.L., Salome, C.M., Yan, K., and Shaw, J. (1982) *Br. J. clin. Pharmacol.* **14**, 464.
Butchers, P.R., Skidmore, I.F., Vardey, C.J., and Wheeldon, A. (1980). *Br. J. Pharmacol.* **71**, 663.
Chen, W.Y. and Chai, H. (1982). *Chest* **81**, 675.
Clarke, J.M., Hamer, J., Shelton, J.R., Taylor, S., and Venning, G.R. (1976). *Lancet* **ii**, 508.
De Vries, K., Goei, J.T., Booy-Noord, H., and Orie, N.G.M. (1962). *Int. Arch. Allergy* **20**, 93.
Fairfax, A.J., McNabb, W.R., Davies, H.J. and Spiro, S.G. (1980). *Thorax* **35**, 526.
FitzGerald, G.A., Barnes, P.J., Hamilton, C., and Dollery, C.T. (1980). *Eur. J. clin. Invest.* **10**, 401.
Goodall, R.J.R., Earis, J.E., Cooper, D.N., Bernstein, A., and Temple, J.G. (1981). *Thorax* **36**, 116.
Grieco, M.H. and Pierson, R.N. (1971). *J. Allergy. clin. Immunol.* **48**, 143.
Hetzel, M.R. (1981). *Thorax* **36**, 481.
Ind, P.W., Barnes, P.J., Brown, M.J., Causon, R., and Dollery, C.T. (1983). *Clin. Allergy* **13**, 61.
Lancet (1982). Editorial. *Lancet* **i**, 1121.
Moore-Ede, M.C., Czeisler, C.A., and Richardson, G.S. (1983). *N. Engl. J. Med.* **309**, 469.
Nadel, J.A. and Barnes, P.J. (1984). *Ann. Rev. Med.* (in press).
Peters, S.P., Schulman, E.S., Schleimer, R.P., Macglashan, D.W., Newball, H.H., and Lichtenstein, L.M. (1982). *Am. Rev. resp. Dis.* **126**, 1034.
Porohecky, L.A. and Wurtman, R.J. (1971). *Pharm Rev.* **23**, 1.
Reinberg, A. and Gervais, P. (1972). *Bull. Physiopath. Res.* **8**, 663.
Reinberg, A., Ghata, J., and Sidi, E. (1963). *J. Allergy* **34**, 323.
Richardson, J.B. (1979). *Am. Rev. resp. Dis.* **119**, 785.
Richardson, J.B. (1981). *Lung* **159**, 315.
Ryan, G., Latimer, K.M., Dolovich, J., and Hargreave, F.E. (1982). *Thorax* **37**, 423.
Skoogh, B.-E. (1983). *Eur. J. resp. Dis.* **64** (suppl 131), 159.
Snashall, P.D., Boother, F.A., and Sterling, G.A. (1978). *Clin. Sci.* **54**, 283.
Soutar, C.A., Carruthers, M., and Pickering, C.A.C. (1977). *Thorax* **32**, 677.
Soutar, C.A., Costello, J., Ijaduola, O., and Turner-Warwick, M. (1975). *Thorax* **30**, 436.
Szentivanyi, A. (1968). *J. Allergy* **42**, 203.
Titinchi, S., Al Shamma, M., Patel, K.R., Kerr, J.W., and Clark, B. (1984). *Clin. Sci.* **66**, 323.
Townshend, M.M. and Smith, A.J. (1973). *Clin. Sci.* **44**, 253.
Ungar, A. and Phillips, J.H. (1983). *Physiol. Rev.* **63**, 787.
Vermeire, P.A. and Vanhoutte, P.M. (1979). *J. appl. Physiol.* **46**, 787.

Discussion

Professor D.C. Flenley

Could the interaction between adrenaline and the vagal system be studied in vagotomized dogs?

Dr P.J. Barnes

These studies are difficult to do *in vivo* because beta agonists change airway smooth muscle tone. Skoogh in Sweden looked at ganglionic neurotransmission in isolated ferret trachea and has shown that beta agonists can reduce cholinergic neurotransmission. More sophisticated techniques measure the activity of nerve cells in airway ganglia and have shown that beta agonists can reduce the propensity of the nerve cells to fire to a depolarizing (excitatory) stimulus. Beta-agonists and adrenaline may therefore have an inhibitory action on ganglia which may be a very important aspect of their beneficial effects. There is no such data yet available on human airways.

Professor C.M. Fletcher

Is there a drop in temperature in hospital wards at night and does warm air prevent a nocturnal drop in peak flow?

Dr P.J. Barnes

In the study to which I referred environmental temperatures were carefully controlled and a fall in core temperature occurred at night, which is independent of the external temperature. However, the temperature drop is very small, but when subjects were given warm, humidified air, to prevent any temperature effect on the airway itself, bronchoconstriction at night was diminished.

Dr G.M. Cochrane

About 20 years ago a series of patients was treated for asthma by vagotomy but clinically this had no effect on nocturnal dips. We have looked at body cooling and airway cooling in hospital and have found two or three patients who respond to maintaining a high core temperature between the hours of 2 and 4 a.m. There are technical difficulties as they have to be almost superheated to prevent their asthma. The airway has to be humidified and we couldn't reproduce the published findings without the patient very nearly drowning in their own secretions.

Dr N. Wilson

I am glad the question of gastro-oesophageal reflux was raised. We studied a group of children with severe asthma by pH monitoring to see whether gastro-oesophageal reflux occurred. It was present in over half of 15 children studied and we were interested in whether this could affect pulmonary function. We measured the PC_{20} to inhaled histamine before and then 90 minutes after drinking dilute hydrochloric acid (0.001 per cent) or placebo in double-blind fashion. In a significant proportion we found that dilute acid caused a very marked increase in their sensitivity to histamine, suggesting that in people with reflux acid in the oesophagus at night can greatly increase their bronchial reactivity. I feel that this is a field that has probably been overlooked.

Dr G.M. Cochrane

This has been studied in adults with gastro-oesosphageal reflux and asthma. If the overnight pH is increased, there is less nocturnal asthma.

Professor D.C. Flenley

What is the effect of ranitidine?

Dr G.M. Cochrane

There was slightly less drop in peak flow, but it didn't cure it.

Dr C.K. Connolly

We have two patients with severe reflux and severe nocturnal dips who have been treated with asilone and, subjectively at least, their nocturnal dips are now less.

Allergic reactions and nocturnal asthma

A. NEWMAN-TAYLOR

Brompton Hospital

Introduction

Worsening of asthmatic symptoms during the nighttime has been recognized as a manifestation of asthma for centuries (Floyer 1698). Serial measurements of lung function in patients with asthma have shown that airway narrowing increases during the nighttime and early morning (Turner-Warwick 1977). It is not surprising that a finger of suspicion should be pointed at the co-habitants of our beds, the house dust mite *D. pteronyssinus*, and nocturnal asthma be attributed to an allergic reaction to the mites in our bedding. However nocturnal asthma occurs as frequently in non-atopic as atopic asthmatics, and there is no convincing evidence to link nocturnal asthma to house-dust mite allergy (Clark and Hetzel 1977).

Nocturnal asthma is probably an exaggeration of the normal circadian variation in airway calibre which reflects airway hyperreactivity characteristic of asthma. Inhalation tests with soluble allergens and low-molecular-weight chemicals may provoke asthmatic reactions which recur on several successive nights and improve spontaneously during the intervening days. The link between these test exposures and nocturnal asthma seems to be increased airway reactivity induced by the 'late' asthmatic reaction.

Nocturnal asthma and airway hyperreactivity

Asthma is now usually defined as narrowing of the airways which varies over short periods of time, either spontaneously or as a result of treatment. A central feature of asthma is airway hyperreactivity — an increased bronchoconstrictor response to non-specific provocative stimuli. Such stimuli include exercise which probably stimulates airway narrowing by evaporative cooling of the airways and inhaled pharmacological agents such as histamine and metacholine. Airway reactivity is commonly and conveniently tested in the laboratory by the response of the airways to the inhalation of increasing concentrations of histamine or metacholine. The degree of airway reactivity is conveniently expressed as the concentration of the stimulus required to provoke a 20 per cent fall in FEV_1 (PC_{20}).

Ryan *et al.* (1982) showed that both the circadian variation in airway calibre and airway responsiveness to inhaled salbutamol are related to the degree of airway reactivity. They studied 39 patients, 27 with current symptoms of asthma, five with a past history of asthma, and nine without asthma, during a period of one week. They found that the greater the degree of airway hyperreactivity, the lower the peak expiratory flow rate on waking in the morning, the greater the difference between the maximum and minimum peak flow rate during the day time, and the greater the response in peak expiratory flow rate to inhaled salbutamol. They also demonstrated that airway reactivity to inhaled histamine was increased in some individuals when FEV_1 was within 10 per cent of the maximum value suggesting that the increased responsiveness to inhaled histamine was not simply a reflection of decreased airway calibre.

Allergen exposure and airway hyperreactivity

Inhalation tests with both soluble allergens, such as grass pollens and house-dust mite, and low-molecular-weight chemicals such as isocyanates, formaldehyde, and plicatic acid, a resin acid of Western Red Cedar, may provoke asthmatic reactions. These may be 'immediate', which develop within minutes of exposure and resolve spontaneously within one or two hours, or 'late' which develop after one or more hours and persist for 24 to 36 hours. In a study of patients with Western Red Cedar asthma, Lam *et al.* (1979) found that in those in whom plicatic acid provoked a 'late' asthmatic reaction, reactivity to inhaled metacholine had increased 24 hours after the test on average 30.8-fold. No increase in airway reactivity occurred at 24 hours post-test in those who had had isolated 'immediate' reactions. Cartier *et al.* (1982) obtained similar results in a study of 12 asthmatic patients in whom asthmatic reactions were provoked by inhalation of soluble allergens. A fall in FEV_1 of greater than 14 per cent occurring between three and eight hours after inhalation test (i.e. 'late' reaction) was associated with a greater than twofold increase in airway reactivity to inhaled histamine which, in several subjects, persisted for more than one week. The severity and duration of increase in airway hyperreactivity, measured as decrease in PC_{20}, was related to the fall in FEV_1 during the 'late' asthmatic reaction. In four patients, PC_{20} remained significantly reduced at times when lung volume measurements—forced expiratory volume in one second, forced vital capacity, total lung capacity, and residual volume — had returned to within 10 per cent of pre-test values. These results suggest that airway reactivity increases as a consequence of the 'late' asthmatic reaction and although this may be attributable in some cases to reduced airway calibre, this is not the explanation in all subjects.

Allergens, airway hyperreactivity, and nocturnal asthma

There are now several reports of recurrent nocturnal asthmatic reactions provoked by a single inhalation of both soluble allergens, including grain (Davies *et al.* 1976) and avian serum protein (Newman Taylor *et al.* 1979), and low-molecular-weight chemicals, including isocyanates (Siracusa *et al.* 1978) and formaldehyde (Newman Taylor *et al.* 1979). In each of these cases, the recurrent nocturnal asthmatic reaction occurred following a late asthmatic reaction. It seems likely that these reactions reflect an exaggeration of the normal circadian variation in airway calibre consequent upon an induced increase in airway reactivity.

Recently Cockroft *et al.* (1984) reported two patients in whom a single exposure to Western Red Cedar provoked recurrent nocturnal asthma. The nocturnal asthma followed a 'late' asthmatic reaction in both cases and was associated with a tenfold reduction in PC_{20} to inhaled histamine which persisted for several days after FEV_1 had returned to pre-test values.

The cause of the induced airway hyperreactivity which follows 'late' asthmatic reactions is unclear. A plausible hypothesis is that it develops as a consequence of inflammation of the airway wall during the late asthmatic reaction. Direct evidence of airway inflammation during the 'late' asthmatic has not been obtained, but local infiltration with neutrophils and eosinophils occurs in the 'late' skin reaction whose time course parallels the airway reaction. Inflammatory cells are probably recruited to the reaction site, either directly or indirectly, by mediators generated by mast cells (Solley *et al*. 1976). Interestingly, 'late' asthmatic reactions are associated with a rise in neutrophil chemotactic activity which is thought to be mast-cell-derived (Nazy *et al*. 1982). Nadel has demonstrated that transient airway reactivity increases in dogs after acute ozone inhalation, and that this is dependent upon neutrophil infiltration of the airway wall (Nadel 1984). Airway reactivity only increased in those dogs in whom neutrophils infiltrated the airway epithelium, and the time course of the neutrophil infiltration paralleled the duration of increase in airway reactivity. Depletion of neutrophils by hydroxyurea treatment prior to ozone inhalation prevented this induced increase in airway reactivity.

References

Cartier, A., Thomson, N.C., Frith, P.A., Roberts, R., and Hargreave, F.E. (1982). *J. Allergy clin. Immunol.* **70**, 170.

Clark, T.J.H. and Hetzel, M.R. (1977). *Bor. J. Dis. Chest* **71**, 87.

Cockroft, D.W., Hoeppner, V.H., and Werner, G.D. (1984). *Clin. Allergy* **14**, 61.

Davies, R.S., Green, M., and Schofield, N.Mc. (1976). *Am. Rev. resp. Dis.* **114**, 1011.

Floyer, J. (1698). *A treatise of the asthma*. Wilkin, London.

Lam, L., Wong, R., and Chan-Yeung, M. (1979). *J. Allergy clin. Immunol.* **70**, 170.

Nadel, J.A. (1984). In *Asthma: physiology, immunopharmacology and treatment*. (ed. A.B. Kay, K.F. Austen, and L.M. Lichtenstein.)

Nadel, J.A. and Davis, B. (1977). In *Asthma: physiology, immunopharmacology and treatment*. (ed. L.M. Lichtenstein and K.F. Austen), p.197. Academic Press, New York.

Nazy, L., Lee, T.H., and Kay, A.B. (1982). *N. Engl. J. Med.* **306**, 497.

Newman-Taylor, A.J., Davies, R.J., Hendrick, D.S., and Pepys, J. (1979). *Clin. Allergy* **9**, 213.

Ryan G., Latimer, K.M., Dolovitch, J., and Hargreave, F.E. (1982). *Thorax* **37**, 423.

Siracusa, A., Curradi, F., and Abbrilli, G. (1978). *Clin. Allergy* **8**, 195.

Solley, G.O., Gleich, G.J., Jordan, R.E., and Schweter, A.L. (1976). *J. clin. Invest.* **58**, 402.

Turner-Warwick, M. (1977). *Br. J. Dis. Chest* **71**, 73.

Discussion

Professor T.J. Clark

Recovery from allergen challenge takes some days, possibly a week or two, and in the study of Platts-Mills and colleagues it took some months before bronchial reactivity returned to normal. Do you have any ideas about the mechanisms underlying this slow recovery of bronchial reactivity after the initial challenge?

Dr A. Newman-Taylor

I suppose that what is happening during the late asthmatic reaction is that there is inflammation occurring within the airway wall. This possibly sets up circuits which take some considerable time to decrease. A study which has been published recently from San Francisco showed that an increase in airway reactivity in a dog model was paralleled by neutrophil infiltration into the airway mucosa. As this resolved over a period of about a month or so, airway reactivity returned to normal. I think my best guess at the present time would be that you are seeing slowly resolving inflammatory changes in airway walls.

Dr P.J. Barnes

So steroids should be the best treatment for nocturnal asthma, but they are not.

Professor D.C. Flenley

Interpretation of the data of Hargreaves and colleagues which you have shown could equally be in terms of having a narrower airway because of a challenge, which then causes a change in PC_{20} for geometric reasons.

Dr A. Newman-Taylor

They looked at four patients where the tests of lung function, including flow rates at low lung volumes, had returned to normal and yet increased airway reactivity persisted for some considerable time after this. One could always say that our tests are not sufficiently sensitive to demonstrate changes in airway calibre.

Dr P.J. Barnes

In that same paper they showed that there was no relationship between PC_{20} and baseline FEV_1.

Dr R.W. Fuller

A recent paper from Chung and co-workers showed that when the initial baseline was reduced with methacholine it had no effect on the PC_{35} for histamine.

Dr A. Newman-Taylor

It suggests that the mechanism which has been suggested is not sufficient to account for the phenomenon of airway hyperreactivity.

Professor M. Turner-Warwick

Dr Hargreaves showed in an earlier paper that PC_{20} did relate to the baseline FEV_1 so the literature is in a muddle.

Dr M. Silverman

Agents other than allergens may induce increased reactivity and induce asthma. Thus food substances, which don't seem to be allergic in their effect, may trigger off increased nocturnal asthma. We have seen children who give a clear history of taking certain foods during the daytime who develop symptoms later at night, which are presumably of non-allergic origin.

Dr A. Newman-Taylor

When I use the word allergen I do not imply that there is an immediate reaction. These reactions may occur with agents such as isocyonates, for which we have no evidence of IgE antibodies.

Dr R.W. Fuller

Do the reactions which you describe recur on subsequent nights, despite avoidance of further exposure and with normal FEV_1 in the intervening day?

Dr A. Newman-Taylor

What I was describing are recurrent nocturnal reactions which I think are a consequence of increased airway reactivity which is persisting during that period of time and is reflected by the increased amplitude of circadian variation.

Clinical implications

T.J. CLARK

Guy's Hospital, London, UK

Deterioration in lung function at night in asthma appears to be largely the result of an increased amplitude in the normal circadian rhythm of airway tone, as demonstrated by cosinor analysis. This worsening of lung function at night appears to be associated with an excess of sudden deaths. Although there does appear to be a significant increase in sudden deaths at night, there is also likely to be an increase during the day as nocturnal asthma is a reflection of bronchial lability, which may predispose to death at any time. Whether better control of the circadian variation in lung function might reduce the incidence of sudden death in asthma remains to be determined. Objective measurements, such as peak flow recording at home, have proved to be very useful in assessment and recognition of nocturnal asthma and may be useful in monitoring patients at risk.

The underlying mechanism of nocturnal asthma is likely to be bronchial hyperreactivity. In patients with normal lung function who are challenged with allergens, this may trigger off nocturnal asthma which may persist for several days after the challenge. The mechanism for this may involve recruitment of neutrophils and inflammatory products into the airway, particularly the airway epithelium. Fluctuation in plasma adrenaline and other factors probably play a permissive role in the pathogenesis of nocturnal wheeze. Other factors, such as gastro-oesophageal reflux may also be important.

The basic aim of treatment is to prevent the worsening of lung function at night and this probably involves the control of bronchial hyperreactivity. Treatment may prove difficult and in some patients a continuous infusion of either ß-agonists or theophylline may fail to prevent the fall in lung function. Inhaled ß-agonists may protect against bronchoconstriction and may work in some patients. Regular inhaled ß-agonist treatment may be sufficient to control symptoms in some patients. Similarly, slow-release theophyllines may also be effective. Corticosteroids, while ineffective in some patients, can control nocturnal symptoms and more studies are needed on the role of inhaled steroids in the treatment of nocturnal asthma, since treatment should be aimed at reducing bronchial hyperreactivity.

Discussion

Dr C.K. Connolly

I disagree that the circadian variation of the normals has anything to do with morning dipping. For a number of reasons the model of a cosinor fitting is totally inappropriate and leads to false conclusions.

Professor T.J. Clark

By using cosinor analysis you can demonstrate a cyclic variation in peak flow in healthy subjects which has the same phase as the cyclic variation in asthmatic subjects. It may be a leap of faith to say that asthma, by having the same phase and a larger amplitude, may be an underdamping of the normal mechanisms. In healthy subjects you can demonstrate some cyclic variation in lung function which has a 24-hour period, and the measurements are highest during the day and lowest during the night. Whether they conform to a sine wave is unimportant.

Professor D.C. Flenley

Most physicists or mathematicians given four points throughout a 24-hour period could fit a sine wave to them. Dr Barnes' data is nothing like a sine wave with a big fall at night which comes back fast. I agree with Dr Barnes that we should try to devise a method of measuring the fall which you try to deduce from your 'non-waking up' studies.

Professor T.J. Clark

The leap of faith is whether normal reactivity and asthmatic reactivity are linked. I certainly wouldn't say that the whole issue hinges on the cyclic variation having a sine wave. Dr Moore-Ede and colleagues have shown a whole variety of functions from sine waves to square waves to little pulses.

Dr P.J. Barnes

I think most people would agree that hyperreactivity amplifies something which may be a circadian rhythm of whatever form.

Professor D.C. Flenley

Is there a cyclical variation in bronchial reactivity?

Dr P.J. Barnes

No, the bronchial reactivity is the same but the underlying mechanism is amplified by the hyperreactivity cycling, although we don't know that the cycling is sinusoidal.

Dr M. Hetzel

It is not correct to say that cosinor analysis is looking at only four points as we measured those four points every day. What the cosinor analysis has shown is that you have the same pattern for a number of days. If you don't try and attempt a mathematical model, you are left with the only other alternative which is pattern recognition. Others have used cosinor analysis with hourly measurements and get the same pattern, but with more accuracy.

The role of beta-adrenoceptor agonists in the treatment of nocturnal asthma

A.J. FAIRFAX

Department of Thoracic Medicine, Staffordshire General Infirmary, Stafford, UK

Introduction

Nocturnal asthma has been observed as a transient phenomenon during recovery from an exacerbation of asthma (Turner-Warwick 1977). It may also occur for several nights following a single bronchial provocation with allergen or other provoking agent (Davies *et al*. 1976; Siracusa *et al*. 1978; Newman-Taylor *et al*. 1979). Repeated nocturnal attacks of asthma occur in many patients with poorly controlled chronic asthma. The importance of the diurnal rhythm of airflow obstruction lies in the fact that asthmatics typically experience their maximal physiological disturbance during sleep in the early hours of the morning when they may be least aware of the severity of their symptoms, when the effects of daytime therapy may have worn off, and at a time when medical assistance is not always readily available.

Adrenoceptor agonists have several different physiological effects all of which may be important in the treatment of asthma. They are known to relax bronchial smooth muscle by stimulation of beta$_2$ receptors. In addition, they may inhibit mast-cell degranulation, have anti-inflammatory properties, increase ciliary motility enhancing mucociliary clearance, and produce vasodilatation (Paterson *et al*. 1979).

In 1984, a wide choice of beta-adrenoceptor agonists is available to the clinician for the treatment of asthma. In general, there has been a swing towards the use of beta$_2$-specific agents. Inhalation has become the preferred route of administration because of its relative effectiveness and lack of side-effects when compared with the oral or intravenous routes (Larsson and Svedmyr 1977). However, the majority of available drugs when given by inhalation produce maximal bronchodilation within one hour of administration and the effect has usually diminished considerably or disappeared altogether by six hours. This time course is inadequate to control nocturnal asthma where the ideal drug, taken at around 22.00–23.00 hours, would produce maximal bronchodilation between 04.00 and 06.00 hours, i.e. have its *peak* effect six to eight hours after administration to coincide with the time of maximal airflow obstruction.

The beta$_2$-specific adrenoceptor agonists regularly administered by inhalation as treatment for asthma include salbutamol, terbutaline, reproterol, pirbuterol, fenoterol, and rimiterol. In the UK oral preparations of all of these compounds except fenoterol and rimiterol are currently available. Oral beta$_2$-specific drugs such as salbutamol have long been recognized to be active for the control of chronic asthma (Epstein *et al.* 1973) although concern has been expressed about the possibility of tachyphylaxis (Jenne 1982). Theoretically, therefore, sustained-release preparations could represent one method of providing effective bronchodilator therapy lasting throughout the night for patients with recurrent nocturnal asthma.

It is instructive to consider some of the possible factors which may determine the occurrence of nocturnal asthma and to review the efficacy of beta-adrenoceptor agonists for overcoming each of these potential mechanisms (Fairfax 1984). They include allergic factors, changes in bronchial hyperreactivity at night, physiological alterations related to sleep and recumbency, the timing of drug administration, and endogenous circadian rhythms, particularly those of circulating catecholamines.

Several controlled clinical trials have attempted to assess the efficacy of oral beta-adrenoceptor agonists for the prevention of nocturnal asthma. The results of these studies will be discussed and the efficacy of the beta$_2$-specific adrenoceptor agonists compared with the protection afforded by other therapeutic agents.

Antiallergic effects

Domestic allergens such as Dermatophagoides pteronyssinus may exacerbate asthma in sensitized subjects, for example in many children and young people (Warner 1976). Bronchial responsiveness to inhaled allergen is increased at night in comparison to during the daytime (Gervais *et al.* 1977). Removal from an environment contaminated by the house dust mite for several weeks has been shown to improve the control of asthma and reduce nocturnal asthma (Platts-Mills *et al.* 1982).

An alternative approach to the problem of house dust mite is to attempt to block allergen-induced bronchospasm pharmacologically. In the laboratory, bronchial allergen challenge commonly produces either an early phase of bronchospasm or an early response with recovery followed by a late reaction which may last throughout the night (Warner 1976). Beta-adrenoceptor agonists are known to have potent antiallergic and mast-cell stabilising effects in skin (Ting *et al.* 1983) and in the lung, an effect partially attributable to their action on beta$_2$-receptors on mast cells (Butchers *et al.* 1980). The early phase of bronchospasm may be readily inhibited by beta$_2$-agonists inhaled before or after allergen inhalation (Orie *et al.* 1973; Pepys and Hutchcroft 1975). The late reaction can be diminished by pre-treatment with sodium cromoglycate, corticosteroids (Booij-Noord *et al.* 1971), or non-steroidal anti-inflammatory drugs (Fairfax *et al.* 1983), but is not inhibited by beta$_2$-specific agonists given before allergen inhalation. Once established, the late phase of bronchospasm is not readily reversed with beta-adrenoceptor agonists (Pepys and Hutchcroft 1975) and this may limit their effectiveness as anti-allergic agents in asthma.

The local concentration of beta$_2$-adrenergic agonist is likely to be important in the modulation of allergic responses and there is doubt as to whether oral preparations can achieve adequate tissue levels to produce this effect. For example, in skin intradermal terbutaline inhibits the allergen-induced wheal-and-flare response but therapeutic doses orally are ineffective (Ting *et al.* 1983). Large doses of oral fenoterol are also ineffective in inhibiting skin allergic reactions (Spector 1978).

As beta-adrenoceptor agonists have the capacity both to inhibit mediator release and to antagonize the effects of mediators, it is possible that the anti-allergic properties of these compounds could contribute to their therapeutic efficacy in nocturnal asthma. Regular exacerbations of asthma during the night are common in patients both with allergic and with 'intrinsic' asthma, where skin and bronchial provocation tests with allergens are negative. Allergen inhalation, including the house-dust mite (Connolly 1981), may therefore not be directly related to the phenomenon of nocturnal asthma and may simply represent one factor ensuring the chronicity of the disorder by increasing bronchial hyperreactivity (Cockcroft *et al.* 1977*a*).

Beta-adrenoceptor agonists and bronchial hyperreactivity

Bronchial hyperreactivity as measured by the responsiveness to inhaled histamine or cholinergic agents (Cockcroft *et al.* 1977*b*) is known to increase at night (De Vries *et al.* 1962). The responsiveness to other non-specific agents such as cold air (O'Byrne *et al.* 1982) is also enhanced (Chen and Chai 1982). It is therefore possible that increased responsiveness of the target organ at night accounts for the phenomenon of nocturnal asthma (Fairfax 1984), this occurring at a time when parasympathetic nervous activity increases, plasma histamine levels rise, and circulating catecholamine levels decrease (Barnes *et al.* 1980). Increased bronchial hyperreactivity may occur for several days after bronchial provocation by inhaled allergen inducing a late phase response (Cockcroft *et al.* 1977*a*). If the diurnal variation of airflow obstruction is an indicator of bronchial hyperreactivity, this mechanism may explain the recurrent nocturnal episodes of asthma which have been reported after some laboratory bronchial provocation tests (Davies *et al.* 1976; Siracusa *et al.* 1978; Newman-Taylor *et al.* 1979).

Do beta-adrenoceptor agonists have a role in reducing bronchial hyperreactivity in asthma, and might this potential effect be beneficial in reducing nocturnal asthma? Both non-selective and selective beta$_2$-agonists when given prior to challenge have been shown to have a direct bronchodilating effect adequate to counteract the bronchoconstrictor effect of inhaled histamine and methacholine. Given by mouth, ephedrine (Spector 1978) and the beta$_2$-specific adrenergic agents such as salbutamol, have been shown to have a significant protective effect (Cockcroft *et al.* 1977*c*). In this study Cockcroft showed that 200 µg of inhaled salbutamol was significantly more effective than 4 mg oral salbutamol which only conferred a weak protective effect on the airway response to histamine. DeVries showed an inhibition by fenoterol (0.08 mg i.m.) in patients with asthma and bronchitis during histamine and, less so, during methacholine challenge (DeVries *et al.* 1982). The effect of beta-adrenoceptor agonists has further been studied by Woolcock and co-workers who demonstrated that the airway dose-response curve to inhaled histamine and methacholine in asthma was shifted to the right by inhaled fenoterol (Salome *et al.* 1983). The duration of the protective effect of fenoterol was followed by repeating the histamine inhalations at different intervals on subsequent days. The shift of the dose-response curve was short-lived and had returned to the untreated position within three hours, i.e. before the bronchodilator action of fenoterol had worn off. The authors suggested that up to 400 µg of inhaled fenoterol every four to five hours would be needed in asthmatics to keep the bronchial responsiveness to histamine within the normal range, a dosing interval which would require patients to be woken during the night.

In the longer term, do regular administrations of beta-adrenoceptor agonists reduce bronchial hyperreactivity? The published data so far do not suggest that chronic administration confers any benefit of this type. For example, Harvey and Tattersfield (1982) gave increasing divided doses of inhaled salbutamol up to 2 mg/day to a group of asthmatics over a four-week period in an attempt to demonstrate tachyphylaxis. This produced no change in the diurnal peak flow pattern and there was no change in either the responsiveness to inhaled histamine or in the acute protection afforded by salbutamol to histamine challenge during the study. Apart from the bronchodilator effect of the beta-adrenoceptor agonists, there does not appear to be any additional benefit on reduction of hyperreactivity to be obtained by regular administration of these drugs in asthma even when they are given by inhalation in large doses to give maximal local concentrations in the bronchial mucosa. In view of the anti-allergic effects of beta-agonists the lack of efficacy in reducing hyperreactivity is, perhaps, surprising. One possible explanation may lie in the lack of efficacy of these agents in inhibiting the late bronchial response to allergen since the latter appears to be an important determinant of hyperreactivity in allergic asthma (Cockcroft et al. 1977a).

Other aetiological factors

Sleep itself appears to be a factor inducing asthma in some subjects (Hetzel and Clark 1979). It is therefore possible that sympathomimetic agents such as ephedrine which alter the level of consciousness and commonly produce insomnia may have a central effect in nocturnal asthma. The use of non-specific beta-adrenoceptor agonists during the night would appear undesirable. Potential adverse effects include cardiac stimulation, induction of arrhythmias, and the elevation of free fatty acid levels. Even the $beta_2$-specific drugs given orally for nocturnal asthma have unnecessary and potentially undesirable effects such as tremor and metabolic actions affecting gluconeogenesis, insulin release, and serum potassium (Taylor et al. 1976). Hypoxaemia is usually maximal at night in asthmatics (Hetzel et al. 1977; Catterall et al. 1982) and adrenoceptor agonists may have the undesirable effect of further decreasing PaO2 (Paterson et al. 1979).

Recumbency at night may encourage gastro-oesophageal reflux, a long-debated possible cause of vagally-mediated asthma. Recent evidence suggests that acid in the oesophagus may produce respiratory changes in asthmatics with oesophagitis in whom the Bernstein test is positive (Davis et al. 1983). In this context it is of interest that $beta_2$-adrenoceptor agonists, such as carbuterol, act as smooth-muscle relaxants decreasing the lower oesophageal sphincter pressure, theoretically making reflux more likely to occur at night (DiMarino and Cohen 1982).

Decreased mucociliary clearance has been demonstrated in mild asthma (Bateman et al. 1983) and clearance is known to decrease during sleep (Bateman et al. 1978). Mucus retention at night is one further factor which could therefore contribute to nocturnal asthma. Adrenoceptor agonists by stimulating mucociliary transport may be beneficial (Paterson et al. 1979) although the rapid reversibility of nocturnal asthma in the morning casts doubt on the importance of mucus plugging at night (Fairfax et al. 1980).

The timing of drug administration may be one further factor enhancing nocturnal asthma. It is currently popular to administer beta-adrenoceptor agonists regularly during the daytime but, as has already been mentioned, few of these agents given by inhalation have an adequate duration of action to maintain bronchodilation throughout the night (Jenne 1981).

Endogenous circadian rhythms

Circadian rhythms which may be relevant to nocturnal asthma include a rise in plasma histamine in the early morning, a fall in plasma cortisol, and a fall in plasma catecholamines and cyclic AMP (Soutar et al. 1977; Mikuni et al. 1978; Barnes et al.

1980). It has been suggested that partial blockade of beta-adrenoreceptors may be the basic abnormality in asthma (Szentivanyi 1968) and a similar mechanism could also account for asthma at night. Carpentiere and co-workers (1983) reported a variable response to inhaled fenoterol given at different times of the day implying changes in beta-receptor responsiveness. Barnes and co-workers (1982), however, found no evidence of beta-adrenoceptor dysfunction at night. These workers have attributed the occurrence of nocturnal asthma to circadian variations of circulating catecholamines both acting directly on the airways and modulating the release of mediators from pulmonary mast cells (Barnes *et al.* 1980; Barnes *et al.* 1982). If this hypothesis were correct, administration of sympathomimetic agents at night would be expected to prevent or even reverse the diurnal airway rhythm. This has not been observed using large doses of oral salbutamol given during the day (Milledge and Morris 1979) or immediately prior to and during sleep (Fairfax *et al.* 1980; Fairfax 1980).

Beta-adrenoceptor agonists in nocturnal asthma

Having considered the potential mechanisms whereby beta-adrenoceptor agonists may influence nocturnal asthma, the question remains as to whether these drugs have a role in clinical practice. Some patients appear to be resistant to the effects of these agents (Fig. 1). Two well-controlled, double-blind clinical trials have studied

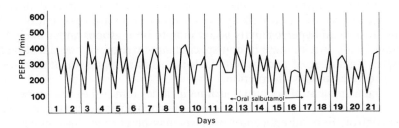

Fig. 1. *Severe nocturnal dips in peak expiratory flow rate in a 29-year-old severe asthmatic showing no improvement with 16 mg slow-release oral salbutamol given before sleep.*

the use of oral slow-release beta$_2$-agonists in nocturnal asthma. In one study (Fairfax *et al.* 1980), 14 chronic asthmatics with regular nocturnal exacerbations were given 16 mg oral slow-release salbutamol before sleep for one week and the results were compared to those with slow-release aminophylline at night and with placebo. Salbutamol produced a significant improvement in morning peak flow rates (mean 251 l/min with salbutamol, 218 l/min with placebo; p <0.01) and the plasma salbutamol levels measured at 06.00 h were similar to those achieved at steady state with a therapeutically effective salbutamol infusion (8 µ/kg/h). The evening peak flow rates were slightly but not significantly improved. Although decreased, the morning dip was not abolished by oral salbutamol and further improvement of morning peak flow was seen in all patients given 200 µg inhaled salbutamol. With this daily dose of salbutamol three of the 14 patients complained of side-effects, namely tremor. The effect of giving 450 mg slow-release aminophylline at night was similar but slightly less effective than salbutamol but the plasma levels of theophylline at 06.00 h using this dosage were sub-optimal.

A similar study was reported by Milledge and Morris (1979). These workers studied the effects of giving a large oral dose of salbutamol over a three-week period to a group of 20 asthmatics with nocturnal exacerbations. The drug was given in a dose of 16 mg both at night and in the morning. With this treatment (which is probably the maximum tolerable for chronic oral administration) 19 per cent of subjects complained of side-effects, mainly trembling of the hands, and only 12 of the group were able to complete the trial. The morning and evening peak flow rates showed a significant improvement but although the 'morning dip' was decreased, it was not abolished despite the large dose of beta$_2$-agonist employed. This casts doubt on the importance of the circadian rhythm of endogenous catecholamines as a prime cause of nocturnal asthma. Aminophylline given orally as a slow-release preparation in a divided dose of 900 mg daily was equally effective in preventing nocturnal asthma but 23 per cent of patients complained of gastric intolerance. Neither drug significantly improved the quality of the night's rest nor decreased the need for concomitant inhaled beta$_2$-agonist therapy. The authors commented that, despite the high incidence of side-effects, it was usually possible to find that individuals would tolerate one or other of the drugs employed.

Conclusions

The control of nocturnal asthma remains a common problem in clinical practice. A diurnal rhythm of airflow obstruction occurs in both intrinsic and extrinsic asthma and allergen exposure is only likely to be important in a proportion of asthmatic patients. Bronchial hyperreactivity is common to both groups and is likely to be an important factor. An increase in non-specific airway reactivity occurs at night, at a time when a number of endogenous factors including parasympathetic tone may further provoke airways obstruction.

The management of nocturnal asthma includes removal of any known provoking factors and therapeutic measures aimed at producing an overall improvement in asthma control. Beta-adrenoceptor agonists may be used in this context and their relative merits in preventing nocturnal asthma are discussed.

Controlled clinical trials have shown a statistical improvement in nocturnal asthma using slow-release salbutamol given either as a single large dose before sleep, or with an additional dose given in the morning. Side-effects are the main limiting factor for oral beta$_2$-adrenoceptor agonists and despite maximal tolerated therapy the diurnal rhythm of airflow obstruction usually persists. This observation casts doubt on the importance of the endogenous circadian rhythm of circulating catecholamines as the principal cause of nocturnal asthma.

References

Barnes, P., FitzGerald, G., Brown, M., and Dollery, C. (1980) *N. Eng. J. Med.* **303**, 263.
Barnes, P.J., Fitzgerald, G.A., and Dollery, C.T. (1982). *Clin. Sci.* **64**, 349.
Bateman, J.R.M., Pavia, D., and Clarke, S.W. (1978). *Clin. Sci.* **55**, 523.
Bateman, J.R.M., Pavia, D., Sheahan, N.F., Agnew, J.E., and Clarke, S.W. (1983). *Thorax* **38**, 463.
Booij-Noord, H., Orie, N.G.M., and De Vries, K. (1971). *J. Allergy clin. Immunol.* **48**, 344.
Butchers, P.R., Skidmore, I.F., Vardey, C.J., and Wheeldon, A. (1980). *Br. J. Pharmacol.* **71**, 663.
Carpentiere, G., Marino, S., and Castello, F. (1983). *Chest* **83**, 211.

Catterall, J.R., Douglas, N.J., Calverley, P.M.A., Brash, H.M., Brezinova, V., Shapiro, C.M., and Flenley, D.C. (1982). *Lancet* **i**, 301.
Chen, W.Y. and Chai, H. (1982). *Chest* **81**, 675.
Cockcroft, D.W., Ruffin, R.E., Dolovich, J., and Hargreave, F.E. (1977*a*). *Clin. Allergy* **7**, 503.
Cockcroft, D.W., Killian, D.N., Mellon, J.J.A., and Hargreave, F.E. (1977*b*). *Clin. Allergy* **7**, 235.
Cockcroft, D.W., Killian, D.N., Mellon, J.J.A., and Hargreave, F.E. (1977*c*). *Thorax* **32**, 429.
Connolly, C.K. (1981). *Respiration* **42**, 258.
Davies, R.J., Green, M., and Schofield, N.M. (1976). *Am. Rev. resp. Dis.* **114**, 1011.
Davis, R.S., Larsen, G.L., and Grunstein, M.M. (1983). *J. Allergy clin. Immunol.* **72**, 393.
De Vries, K., Goei, J.T., Booij-Noord, H., and Orie, N.G.M. (1962). *Int. Arch. Allergy* **20**, 93.
De Vries, K., Gokemeyer, G.H., Koeter, J.G.R., Monchy, J.G.R. de., Bork, L.E. van., Kauffman, H.F., and Meurs, H. (1982). In *Perspectives in Asthma 1. Bronchial Hyperreactivity* (ed. J. Morley), p.107. Academic Press, London.
DiMarino, A.J. and Cohen, S. (1982). *Digest. Dis. Sci.* **27**, 1063.
Epstein, S.W., Barnard, J.A., and Zsoter, T.T. (1973). *Am. Rev. resp. Dis.* **108**, 1367.
Fairfax, A.J. (1980). *N. Engl. J. Med.* **303**, 1300.
Fairfax, A.J. (1984) *Res. Clin. Forums* **4**.
Fairfax, A.J., Hanson, J.M., and Morley, J. (1983). *Clin. exp. Immunol.* **52**, 393.
Fairfax, A.J., McNabb, W.R., Davies, H.J., and Spiro, S.G. (1980). *Thorax* **35**, 526.
Gervais, P., Reinberg, A., Gervais, C., Smolensky, M., and de France, O. (1977). *J. Allergy clin. Immunol.* **59**, 207.
Harvey, J.E. and Tattersfield, A.E. (1982). *Thorax* **37**, 280.
Hetzel, M.R., Clark, T.J.H., and Houston, K. (1977). *Thorax* **32**, 418.
Hetzel, M.R. and Clark, T.J.H. (1979). *Thorax* **34**, 749.
Jenne, J.W. (1981). *Lung* **159**, 295.
Jenne, J.W. (1982). *J. Allergy clin. Immunol.* **70**, 413.
Larsson, S. and Svedmyr, N. (1977). *Am. Rev. resp. Dis.* **116**, 861.
Mikuni, M., Saito, Y., Koyama, T., Daiguji, M., Yamashita, I., Honma, M., and Ui, M. (1978). *Life Sci.* **22**, 667.
Milledge, J.S. and Morris, J. (1979). *J. int. Med. Res.* **7** (suppl. 1), 106.
Newman-Taylor, A.J., Davies, R.J., Hendrick, D.J. and Pepys, J. (1979). *Clin. Allergy* **9**, 213.
O'Byrne, P.M., Ryan, G., Morris, M., McCormack, D., Jones, N.L., Morse, J.L.C., and Hargreave, F.E. (1982). *Am. Rev. resp. Dis.* **125**, 281.
Orie, N.G.M., Campagne, J.G.V.L., Knol, K., Booij-Noord, H. and De Vries, K. (1973). In *Intal in bronchial asthma* (ed. J. Pepys and Y. Yamamura). 8th International Congress of Allergology, Tokyo.
Paterson, J.W., Woolcock, A.J., and Shenfield, G.M. (1979). *Am. Rev. resp. Dis.* **120**, 1149.
Pepys, J. and Hutchcroft, B.J. (1975). Bronchial provocation tests in etiologic diagnosis and analysis of asthma. *Am. Rev. resp. Dis.* **112**, 829.
Platts-Mills, T.A.E., Tovey, E.R., Mitchell, E.B., Moszoro, H., Nock, P. and Wilkins, S.R. (1982). *Lancet* **2**, 675.
Salome, C.M., Schoeffel, R.E., Yan, K., and Woolcock, A.J. (1983). *Thorax* **38**, 854.
Siracusa, A., Curradi, F., and Abbritti, G. (1978). *Clin. Allergy* **8**, 195.
Soutar, C.A., Carruthers, M., and Pickering, C.A.C. (1977). *Thorax* **32**, 677.
Spector, S.L. (1978). *Chest* **73**, (Suppl.), 976.
Szentivanyi, A. (1968). *J. Allergy* **42**, 203.
Taylor, M.W., Gaddie, J., Murchison, L.E., and Palmer, K.N.V. (1976). *Br. Med. J.* **1**, 22.
Ting, S., Zweiman, B., and Lavker, R. (1983). *J. Allergy clin. Immunol.* **71**, 437.
Turner-Warwick, M. (1977). *Br. J. Dis. Chest* **71**, 73.
Warner, J.O. (1976). *Arch. Dis. Child* **51**, 905.

Discussion

Professor T.J. Clark

Even having swallowed enough salbutamol to make patients shake all night or enough aminophylline there is a good response to an inhaled beta-agonist first thing in the morning. I think one has to realize that with oral therapy, particularly with xanthines, patients are titrated to accept the maximum tolerable dose and even two tablets are unable to bring them up to really therapeutic levels, whereas with inhaled therapy it is usually two puffs. There is good evidence that if you increase the dose of inhaled therapy, which has a very much wider safety margin, you might be having a different result than using low-dose inhaled therapy. You can also get a more prolonged action by taking a higher inhaled dose.

Dr A. Fairfax

I think there are a number of possible explanations for the greater effect of inhaled rather than oral beta-agonists. One may be the local effect at the receptor organ in the bronchus, and there is a disparity between the anti-allergic effects of these drugs given topically in the skin and the lack of effects when they are given by mouth. Also there is a lack of effect on histamine challenge when they are given by mouth, whereas they are highly effective on inhibiting histamine and methacholine challenge when given by inhalation. This may all be explained by a local concentration effect but on the other hand it may be something much more subtle. It may be that a sudden stimulus is much more effective than continuous steady-state stimulus. We were producing high but sustained levels of salbutamol overnight that were not protecting these patients, and yet they were responsive to the drug when given by inhalation. Obviously oral drugs are second best to inhaled because of the lack of efficacy by the oral route of the drugs we have in comparison to the inhaled drugs, but I think we need a drug which has a peak effect between six and eight hours after administration, not the tail end of the effect.

Dr D.J. Lane

Ann Woolcock showed that she could alter bronchial hyperreactivity with inhaled fenoterol but not with an oral dose, yet when treating nocturnal asthma we use oral drugs because we believe we can't give the inhaled drug through to the appropriate time in the morning.

Dr A. Fairfax

I think the evidence is that we are just getting a bronchodilator effect that is lasting over night.

Dr P.J. Barnes

There is a very convincing study by Sandy Anderson from Sydney who showed that oral beta-agonists have no protection against exercise-induced asthma whereas inhaled beta-agonists given in a dose that gives exactly the same bronchodilatation completely protect against it, so obviously there is a big difference for the same dose that reaches the beta receptors on the smooth muscle. Presumably there are surface cells, luminal mast cells or airway epithelial cells.

Professor M. Turner-Warwick

If you have a 'morning dipper' and instead of giving them inhaled salbutamol you infuse them with salbutamol, presumably it will not be effective?

Dr A. Fairfax

It will decrease their fall in peak flow but it won't abolish it.

Professor M. Turner-Warwick

And if you just give it at 6 o'clock in the morning?

Dr P.J. Barnes

In our studies which were with infused adrenaline in the early morning it did reverse the fall in peak flow, in people who had labile airway obstruction.

Dr A. Fairfax

You gave an acute short-term infusion of adrenaline at 4 a.m. but we gave an over-night infusion.

Professor D.C. Flenley

How did they sleep?

Dr A. Fairfax

They all went to sleep over night. Four of the 14 complained of tremor, and one became euphoric on one of these infusions. In high doses beta-agonists, even the beta$_2$-specific ones, do have a central stimulant effect.

Dr J.G. Ayres

We have recently studied four patients with severe asthma with continuous subcutaneous infusions of terbutaline, not just over night or for 24 hours, but for days and weeks at home. These four patients, who were previously refractory to massive doses of steroids inhaled by nebuliser and to salbutamol in a dose of 50 mg daily, have been controlled with relatively small doses of terbutaline; in two patients with 1 mg daily and in two who were predominantly 'morning dippers' with 12 mg daily. These patients were getting shakes on nebulised salbutamol treatment, but with subcutaneous treatment have no apparent side-effects. I cannot explain this.

The role of theophylline in the management of asthma

A. GREENING

City Hospital, Edinburgh, UK

One of the commonest and best reported remedies of asthma ... is strong coffee. To the question, 'Have you tried strong coffee?' the asthmatic is pretty sure to answer 'Yes', and he is also pretty sure to add that it gives him relief. ... The *rationale* of its efficacy is, I think, to be found, on the one hand, in the physiological effects of coffee ..., and, on the other, in a feature in the clinical history of asthma which I have long observed ... This fact is that *sleep favours asthma* — that spasm of the bronchial tubes is more prone to occur during the insensibility and lethargy of sleep than during the waking hours. [Hyde Salter 1859]

Introduction

Although Dr Salter recognized the benefit of methylxanthine-containing beverages in the management of asthma one and a quarter centuries ago, it took 80 years for the specific introduction of theophylline in the management of acute, severe asthma (Herrman *et al*. 1937) and c. 120 years to appreciate the advantages of sustained-release theophylline preparations in the management of nocturnal asthma. The narrow therapeutic index of theophyllines has been a major factor in hitherto limiting their clinical use, at least in the United Kingdom. However, the advent of convenient, reliable theophylline assays (Soldin and Hill 1977; Ishizaki *et al*. 1979) and sustained-release preparations (Weinberger *et al*. 1978; Spangler *et al*. 1978), together with information on the pharmacokinetics (Jenne *et al*. 1972; Hendeles *et al*. 1978) has recently encouraged much increased, and more rational, use. Nevertheless, the large variation between individuals in dose requirements (Jenne *et al*. 1972; Greening *et al*. 1981), in conjunction with the narrow therapeutic index, means that to obtain maximum clinical benefit the physician needs to be particularly aware of the factors influencing drug metabolism.

Mechanisms of action of theophylline

Prior to considering the metabolism and pharmacokinetics of theophylline preparations for application in the management of nocturnal asthma, it is worth reflecting on the mechanism of action of these drugs.

In 1962, Butcher and Sutherland reported that theophylline, *in vitro*, inhibited phosphodiesterase resulting in an increase in intracellular adenosine 3', 5'-cyclic monophosphate (cAMP). At the same time the importance of cAMP in regulating smooth muscle tone was recognized. The view thus became firmly established, and it is still quoted in many textbooks, that theophylline exerts its bronchodilator effects via phosphodiesterase inhibition. More recent data, however, must raise serious doubts as to the validity of this view. Polson *et al.* (1978) showed that theophylline concentrations at the upper end of the 'therapeutic range' produced only about 10 per cent inhibition of phosphodiesterase activity in broken cell preparations of human lung tissue. Further the effective phosphodiesterase inhibitor, dipyridamole, appears to have no bronchodilator activity (Ruffin and Newhouse 1981). Alternative mechanisms of action have been proposed. Horrobin *et al.* (1977) suggested that methylxanthines may act as prostaglandin antagonists, though their observations on a perfused rat mesenteric artery preparation require additional data before their conclusions can be extended to human bronchial muscle. Kolbeck and colleagues (1979), using guinea-pig tracheal rings and dog tracheal muscle strips, demonstrated that theophylline at 9 μg ml^{-1} 5 x 10^{-5}M) resulted in 50 per cent muscle relaxation, cellular uptake of calcium and subcellular redistribution of elemental calcium consistent with sequestration of calcium in mitrochondria and a decrease in myoplasmic calcium ion concentration.

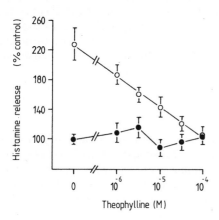

Fig. 1. Histamine release from rat mast cells stimulated with calcium ionophore, 0.3 μg/ml^{-1}. Histamine release was enhanced by 10-min preincubation with adenosine, 10 μm. The inhibition of this enhancement by theophylline, 10^{-6} to 10^{-4}M, is shown by the open circles (○). Theophylline, in the absence of adenosine (●) exerts no influence on ionophore-induced histamine release. (Adapted from Marquardt et al. (1978).)

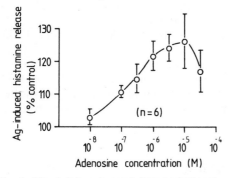

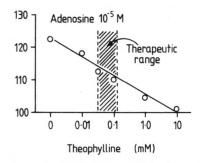

Fig. 2. The left-hand panel demonstrates the dose-dependent enhancement by adenosine of antigen-induced histamine release from rat mast cells. The right-hand panel indicates the inhibition of adenosine (10^{-5}M) enhanced, antigen-induced histamine release, by theophylline at various concentrations. The conventional therapeutic range of plasma theophylline is indicated by the shaded area. (Adapted from Fredholm and Sydbom (1980).)

However, the proposition that this author considers most interesting is that theophyllines may be acting as antagonists of endogenous adenosine. The recognition of adenosine antagonism by theophylline is not new (Ally and Nakatsu 1976) and several cell types have adenosine receptors (Fox and Kelly 1978). Histamine release from rat mast cells, stimulated by anti-IgE, concanavalin-A, and calcium ionophere (Marquardt *et al.* 1978) or by antigen (Fredholm and Sydbom 1980), is enhanced by adenosine, the effect of which is inhibited by theophylline in the range 10^{-6}–10^{-4} M (Figs. 1 and 2). Adenosine also appears to cause relaxation of isolated animal airways, whose tone has been artificially increased (Coleman 1976; Farmer and Farrar 1976). Finally, in patients inhaled adenosine causes a dose-dependent reduction in airways conductance (Cushley *et al.* 1983), bronchoconstriction being maximal within five minutes (Fig. 3). The evidence, therefore, that theophyllines exert their effects via antagonism of endogenous adenosine is circumstantial but attractive.

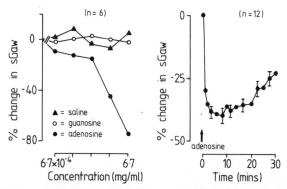

Fig. 3. *The left-hand panel demonstrates the dose-dependent reduction in airways conductance by inhaled adenosine for six allergic asthmatic subjects. Inhaled guanosine and saline had no effect. The right-hand panel indicates the time course of bronchoconstriction induced by a single inhalation of adenosine. The points represent the mean ± SEM percentage change in sGaw, from baseline, for twelve asthmatic subjects. (Adapted from Cushley* et al. *(1983).)*

Theophyllines may influence asthma by mechanisms other than bronchodilation. They can improve diaphragmatic contractibility (Aubier *et al.* 1981) (though this may be more relevant to acute, severe asthma). They may affect airway inflammation, via effects on neutrophil chemotaxis (Tse *et al.* 1972) and degranulation (Zurier *et al.* 1974). Finally, and perhaps of most relevance to nocturnal asthma, they may influence mucociliary clearance. Aminophylline infusion can improve mucociliary clearance (Matthys and Köhler 1980) and mucociliary clearance is reduced in asthma (Bateman *et al.* 1979) and at night (Bateman *et al.* 1978). Data on the effects of theophylline on nocturnal mucociliary clearance in asthma, however, are lacking.

Plasma theophylline levels

Mitenko and Ogilvie (1973), using incremental doses of intravenous theophylline, demonstrated a dose-response relationship between plasma theophylline concentration and reversal of airflow obstruction in asthma (Fig. 4). However, their relatively small improvements in FEV_1 at plasma concentrations less than 10 μg ml⁻¹ gave objective support to the earlier evidence (Turner-Warwick 1957) on symptomatic improvements, that 10 μg ml⁻¹ was the lower end of a 'therapeutic range'. The upper end is arbitrarily taken as 20 μg ml⁻¹, leaving a 'safety margin' to levels where serious

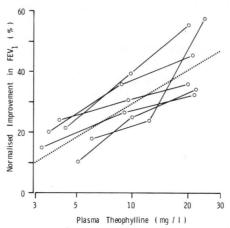

Fig. 4. The dose–response relationship for changes in FEV_1, against plasma theophylline concentration. The individual data for six asthmatic subjects are shown. (Adapted from Mitenko and Ogilvie (1973).)

toxic effects, such as convulsions and cardiac arrhythmias, might ensue (Zwillich *et al.* 1975; Jacobs *et al.* 1976). Adverse, but not dangerous effects such as nausea, abdominal discomfort or headache occur more frequently with plasma levels above 20 μg ml⁻¹ (Hendeles and Weinberger 1980) although some patients experience them at much lower levels (Greening *et al.* 1981).

Using sustained-release theophylline preparations it is possible to achieve plasma levels within this 'therapeutic range' throughout the night (*vide infra*), though careful consideration should be made of factors that may affect drug clearance so as to avoid overdosing.

Theophylline metabolism

Theophylline is extensively metabolized in the liver by dealkylation and hydroxylation. Less than 10 per cent is excreted unchanged in the urine (Jenne *et al.* 1976) (the urinary metabolites being 3-methylxanthine, 1, 3-dimethyluric acid, and 1-methyluric acid) (Jenne *et al.* 1976). In rats, phenobarbital which causes induction of the hepatic P-450 cytochrome and 3-methylcholanthrene which induces formation of a modified cytochrome, P¹-450 (also known as P-448), both increase theophylline metabolism (Lohman and Miech 1976) (though in humans the P¹-450 system may be the more important). Many of the factors that have been observed clinically to alter theophylline metabolism, are almost certainly operating via effects on the hepatic microsomes, e.g. liver disease (Jusko *et al.* 1977), cigarette smoke (Powell *et al.* 1977) (presumably due to polycyclic hydrocarbons such as 3-methylcholanthrene and 3, 4-benzpyrene), and drugs (cimetidine (Reitberg *et al.* 1981), sulphinpyrazone (Birkett *et al.* 1983)).

Theoretically, diet too may affect theophylline metabolism since high-protein diets are said to stimulate the cytochrome P^1-450/P-448 system, (Kappas *et al*. 1976), and indeed high-protein diets are found to result in lower plasma theophylline levels (Kappas *et al*. 1976; Feldman *et al*. 1980; Thompson *et al*. 1983). However, the effects of dietary components upon drug absorption rather than direct influence on metabolism have been proposed (Thompson *et al*. 1983) as an alternative explanation.

In the circulation theophylline appears to bind almost exclusively to albumin (Buss *et al*. 1983) and is about 40 per cent bound (Buss *et al*. 1983). Thus, in hypoalbuminaemic states (e.g. liver disease) plasma theophylline levels could be misleading since more of the drug will be in an unbound (and therefore active) state.

Nocturnal pharmacokinetics of theophylline

There are a number of reports that indicate temporal variations in plasma theophylline (Kyle *et al*. 1980) and reduced clearance at night in adults (Thompson *et al*. 1983) and in children (Scott *et al*. 1981) (Fig. 5(a)). However other well-

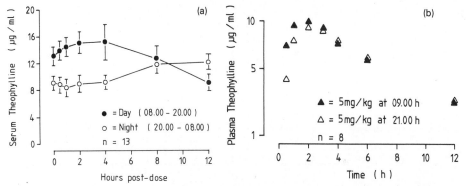

Fig. 5.(a) Comparison of diurnal (●) and nocturnal (○) serum theophylline concentrations for 13 subjects studied during two consecutive dosing intervals. (Adapted from Scott et al. *(1981).) (b) Comparison of diurnal (▲) and nocturnal (△) plasma theophylline concentrations for eight subjects following an oral dose of theophylline, 5mg/kg. Investigations were separated by a seven-day interval and followed a 12 h fast; nor was food permitted for 2.4 h following drug administration. (Adapted from Taylor* et al. *(1983).)*

controlled studies have found no differences between the diurnal and nocturnal disposition of the drug (Taylor *et al*. 1983) (Fig. 5(b)). It seems likely that some of these discrepancies can be accounted for by diurnal variation in dietary intake and consequent differences in drug absorption. An alternative but intriguing explanation is that posture influences plasma theophylline concentrations. Warren *et al*. (1983) found that following intravenous infusion of theophylline the mean peak theophylline concentration was significantly higher with subjects upright than when supine (18.3 vs. 12.4 µg ml⁻¹).

Clinical trials of theophyllines in the management of nocturnal asthma

The introduction of sustained-release preparations have made a considerable difference to the efficacy of theophyllines in the control of nocturnal asthma. Early studies with sustained-release aminophylline indicated significant reductions of the nocturnal fall in FEV_1 (Cole and Al-Khader 1979) or PEFR (Milledge and Morris 1979) when compared with placebo. A more comprehensive trial, by Fairfax and colleagues (1980), comparing sustained-release aminophylline to sustained-release salbutamol and placebo, found that five out of 14 patients achieved a significant reduction in the nocturnal PEFR fall. However, this investigation highlights the importance of using the correct dose of drug, and plasma theophylline levels six hours post-dosage (i.e. not far from the peak levels) indicated that only three patients achieved a level above 10 µg ml^{-1} and all nine non-responders had low levels (mean 6.3 µg ml^{-1}), five having levels of 5µg ml^{-1}. It is likely, therefore, that the lack of clinical benefit was related to inadequate dose of drug. The value of achieving adequate blood levels is exemplified by the work of Barnes *et al.* (1982) who found that sustained-release aminophylline when used in a dose that gave trough (10 h post-dose) theophylline levels of 10.9 ± 0.6 (range 8–15) µg ml^{-1}, completely abolished the nocturnal fall in PEFR (Fig. 6) for 12 of 12 mild-to-moderate asthmatics (two of the 12 also responded to placebo). In addition all patients reported a subjective

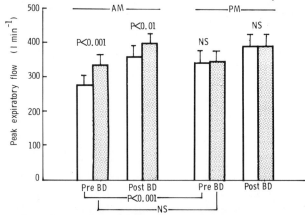

Fig. 6. Mean peak expiratory flow (± SEM) for 12 asthmatic patients following placebo (open bars) or active (slow-release aminophylline, 10.9 mg/kg; stippled bars) at 23.00 h. Values before and after bronchodilator (BD; salbutamol 200 µg in the morning and evening) are shown. Active treatment completely abolished the fall in morning PEF (compare a.m. and p.m. pre-BD panels). Responsiveness to inhaled salbutamol was maintained (compare a.m. and pre-BD and post-BD panels). (Reproduced with permission from Barnes et al. (1982).)

improvement while on active drug and the use of inhaled salbutamol during the night was significantly less than when on placebo (per two weeks; 2.0 ± 1.0 vs. 8.7 ± 1.6 metered doses). The dose of aminophylline required to achieve these results was greater than that conventionally prescribed (range 550–775 mg; which calculated on mg/kg body weight was 9.1–11.4; mean ± SEM 10.4 ± 0.2 mg/kg), but it should be emphasized that this represented the *single* dose of drug given over a 24-hour period.

Although asthmatics can be symptomatically and objectively improved with appropriate doses of sustained-release theophyllines, and appear to experience no unwanted drug effects, there may be some theoretical concern that the central stimulatory effects of the drug could cause insomnia or sleep disturbance. Objective data concerning this point are few. Preliminary work by Rhind *et al.* (1984) finds that sustained-release choline theophyllinate can significantly reduce nocturnal falls in FEV_1 of mild-to-moderate asthmatics and give good symptomatic relief. At the same time EEG monitoring of sleep times and stages suggests that, when on the active preparation, total sleep time was reduced (306 ± 78 min vs. placebo 348 ± 48 min; $p<.05$) and there was an increase in intervening wakefulness and drowsiness.

Nevertheless, these patients thought they had slept better while on the active drug, rather than placebo. It may prove necessary to consider possible long-term effects of drug-induced mild sleep deprivation. Alternatively, the adequate treatment of nocturnal asthma may result in better 'true' sleep quality.

Nocturnal asthma and theophyllines: a personal view

Theophyllines are more demanding in their prescription than most of the drugs used in the management of asthma, because of their narrow 'therapeutic index' and the various influences in their metabolism. However, when correctly used, the therapeutic benefits in the management of nocturnal asthma are most rewarding. As yet, there are no reports in the literature to suggest that any other form of therapy is as effective as sustained-release theophylline preparations. Therefore, the avoidance of treatment with theophyllines because they are 'too dangerous' or 'too difficult' to use may mean depriving some asthmatics of a very valuable form of therapy for their troublesome or distressing nocturnal symptoms. The vast majority of patients with asthma have only mild-to-moderate disease that is readily controlled in the daytime by inhaled $ß_2$-agonists. A significant proportion of these patients will also have nocturnal symptoms of varying severity. For those with regular nocturnal problems a single dose of a sustained-release theophylline preparation, taken on retiring to bed, can be a very effective form of therapy. Ideally, the dose for each patient should be checked by plasma theophylline levels. In practice one often aims to 'underdose' a little and only increase the dose, guided by plasma levels, if adequate symptomatic relief is not obtained. In the absence of factors that affect theophylline metabolism, a single daily dose of sustained-release aminophylline, 9.0 mg/kg (approximately equivalent to 7.5 mg/kg *theophylline*) should avoid 'toxic' plasma levels, but will underdose quite a number of patients. Therapy is perhaps easiest to apply if the physician familiarizes himself with one or possibly two formulations and restricts his prescribing habits to these. One should also remain aware of the multitude of theophylline preparations available (*Lancet* 1983), several of which are compound preparations and make sure that patients are not inadvertently taking more than one preparation.

References

Ally, A.I. and Nakatsu, K. (1976). *J. Pharmacol. exp. Ther.* **199**, 208.
Aubier, M., De Troyer, A., and Sampson, M. (1981). *N. Engl. J. Med.* **305**, 249.
Barnes, P.J., Greening, A.P., Neville, L., Timmers, J., and Poole, G.W. (1982). *Lancet* **i**, 299.
Bateman, J.R.M., Pavia, D., Sheahan, N.F., Agnew, J.E., and Clarke, S.W. (1979). *Thorax* **34**, 418.
Bateman, J.R.M., Pavia, D., and Clarke, S.W. (1978). *Clin. Sci. Molec. Med.* **55**, 523.
Birkett, D.J., Miners, J.O., and Attwood, J. (1983). *Br. J. clin. Pharmacol.* **15**, 567.
Buss, D., Leopold, D., Smith, A.P., and Routledge, P.A. (1983). *Br. J. clin. Pharmacol.* **15**, 399.
Butcher, R.W. and Sutherland, E.W. (1962). *J. Biol. Chem.* **237**, 1244.
Cole, R.B. and Al-Khader, A. (1979). *J. int. Med. Res.* **7** (Suppl. 1), 40.
Coleman, R.A. (1976). *Br. J. Pharmacol.* **57**, 51.
Cushley, M.J., Tattersfield, A.E., and Holgate, S.T. (1983). *Br. J. clin. Pharmacol.* **15**, 161.
Fairfax, A.J., McNabb, W.R., Davies, H.J. and Spiro, S.G. (1980). *Thorax* **35**, 526.
Farmer, J.B. and Farrar, D.G. (1976). *J. Pharm. Pharmacol.* **28**, 748.

Feldman, C.H., Hutchison, V.E., Pippenger, C.E., Blumenfeld, T.A., Feldman, B.R., and Davis, W.J. (1980). *Pediatrics* **66**, 956.
Fox, I.H. and Kelly, W.N. (1978). *Ann. Rev. Biochem.* **47**, 655.
Fredholm, B.B. and Sydbom, A. (1980). *Agents Actions* **10**, 145.
Greening, A.P., Baillie, E., Gribbin, H.R., and Pride, N.B. (1981). *Thorax* **36**, 303.
Hendeles, L. and Weinberger, M. (1980). *Eur. J. resp. Dis.* **61** (suppl. 109), 103.
Hendeles, L., Weinberger, M., and Bighley, L. (1978). *Am. Rev. resp. Dis.* **118**, 97.
Herrman, G., Aynesworth, M.B., and Martin, J. (1937). *J. Lab. clin. Med.* **23**, 135.
Horrobin, D.F., Manku, M.S., Franks, D.J., and Hamet, P. (1977). *Prostaglandins* **13**, 33.
Ishizaki, T., Wantanabe, M., and Morishita, M. (1979). *Br. J. clin. Pharmacol.* **7**, 333.
Jacobs, M.H., Senior, R.M., and Kessler, G. (1976). *J. Am. med. Ass.* **235**, 1983.
Jenne, J.W., Nagasawa, H.T., and Thompson R.D. (1976). *Clin. Pharmacol. Ther.* **19**, 375.
Jenne, J.W., Wyze, E., Rood, F.S., and MacDonald, F.M. (1972). *Clin. Pharmacol. Therap.* **13**, 349.
Jusko, W.J., Kroup, J.R., Vance, J.W., Schentag, J.J., and Kuritzky, P. (1977). *Ann. intern. Med.* **86**, 400.
Kappas, A., Anderson, K.E., Conney, A.H., and Alvares, A.P. (1976). *Clin. Pharmacol. Ther.* **20**, 643.
Kolbeck, R.C., Spier, W.A., Carrier, G.O., and Bransome, E.D. (1979). *Lung* **156**, 173.
Kyle, G.M., Smolensky, M.H., Thorne, L.G., Hsi, B.P., Robinson, A., and McGovern, J.P. (1980). In *Recent advances in the chronobiology of allergy and immunology* (ed. M.H. Smolensky, A. Reinberg, and J.P. McGovern), p.95. Pergamon Press, Oxford.
Lancet (1983). Editorial. *Lancet* **ii**, 607.
Lohmann, S.M., and Miech, R.P. (1976). *J. Pharmacol. exp. Ther.* **196**, 213.
Marquardt, D.L., Parker, C.W., and Sullivan, T.J. (1978). *J. Immunol.* **120**, 871.
Matthys, H., and Köhler, (1980). *Eur. J. resp. Dis.* **61** (Suppl. 109), 98.
Milledge, J.S. and Morris, J. (1979). *J. int. Med. Res.* **7** (suppl. 1), 106.
Mitenko, P.A. and Ogilvie, R.I. (1973). *N. Engl. J. Med.* **289**, 600.
Polson, J.B., Krzanowski, J.J., Goldman, A.L., and Szentivanyi, A. (1978). *Clin. exp. Pharmacol. Physiol.* **5**, 535.
Powell, J.R., Thiercelin, J.F., Vozeh, S., Sansom, L., and Riegelman, S. (1977). *Am. Rev. resp. Dis.* **116**, 17.
Reitberg, D.P., Bernhard, H., and Schentag, J.J. (1981). *Ann. intern. Med.* **95**, 582.
Rhind, G.B., Connaughton, J.J., McFie, J., Douglas, N.J., and Flenley, D.C. (1984). *Am. Rev. resp. Dis.* (Abstr.) (in press).
Ruffin, R.E. and Newhouse, M.T. (1981). *Eur. J. resp. Dis.* **62**, 123.
Salter, H. (1859). *Edinb. med. J.* **IV**, 1109.
Scott, P.H., Tabachnik, E., MacLeod, S., Correia, J., Newth, C., and Levison, H. (1981). *J. Pediat.* **99**, 476.
Soldin, S.J. and Hill, J.G. (1977). *Clin. Biochem.* **10**, 74.
Spangler, D.L., Kaloff, D.D., Bloom, F.L., and Witty, H.J. (1978). *Ann. Allergy* **40**, 6.
Taylor, D.R., Duffin, D., Kinney, C.D., and McDevitt, D.G. (1983). *Br. J. Clin. Pharmacol.* **16**, 413.
Thompson, P.J., Skypala, I., Dawson, S., McAllister, W.A.C., and Turner-Warwick, M. (1983). *Br. J. Clin Pharmacol.* **16**, 267.
Tse, R.L., Phelps, P., and Urban, D. (1972). *J. Lab. clin. Med.* **80**, 264.
Turner-Warwick, M. (1957). *Br. med. J.* **3**, 67.
Warren, J.B., Turner, C., Dalton, N., Thomson, A., Cochrane, G.M., and Clark, T.J.H. (1983). *Br. J. clin. Pharmacol.* **16**, 405.
Weinberger, M., Hendeles, L., and Bighley, L. (1978). *N. Engl. J. Med.* **299**, 852.
Zurier, R.B., Weissman, G., Hoffstein, S., Kammerman, S., and Tai, H.H. (1974). *J. clin. Invest.* **53**, 297.
Zwillich, C.W., Sutton, F.D., Neff, T.A., Cohns, W.M., Matthay, R.A., and Weinberger, M. (1975). *Am. intern. Med.* **82**, 784.

Discussion

Dr D. Pavia

We have administered theophyllines to asthmatic patients to ascertain whether we could improve the reduction in mucociliary clearance at night which we have observed. In a pilot study on four asthmatics who were given 450 mg b.d. for one week, then crossed over with a placebo double-blind, there was a 50 per cent improvement in the clearance during the night when on theophylline compared to the placebo. These are results of small numbers and seemed to be mainly contributed by two out of the four patients.

Dr P.J. Barnes

Do you have data on beta-agonists given in the same way?

Dr D. Pavia

We have no data at night on beta-agonists being given to asthmatics.

Other Drugs

M.R. HETZEL

Whittington and University College Hospitals, London, UK

Introduction

Willis (1679) comments on nocturnal asthma that 'There is scarce anything more sharp or terrible than the fits thereof'. This is equally true today and, in more severe cases, nocturnal asthma still represents a formidable therapeutic challenge. Sixteenth-century asthma patients would no doubt have found modern drugs vastly preferable to the 'Foetid gums, musk, vitriolic ether and opium' recommended by Willis but today's clinician, like Willis, is obliged to use several drugs, often with significant toxicity, in his attempts to control more refractory cases of nocturnal asthma.

In the management of nocturnal asthma there are three broad areas of therapeutic approach — if one accepts the premise that it results from the combined effects of a normal circadian rhythm in airway calibre which is amplified by the asthmatic's excessive bronchial lability. First, one could 'stop the clock' and remove the rhythmic stimulus to bronchoconstriction. A major problem here is that the biological clock driving the rhythm in airway calibre is largely unidentified at present; although there is reason to believe that the main biological clock driving all circadian rhythms is situated in the hypothalamus. There are no drugs currently available which could switch off the clock and, if there were, the side-effects of such treatment might be considerable since many important rhythms, for example the rhythm in sleep and wakefulness, might also be affected. It is, nevertheless, possible to inhibit the clock by other means. It is normally synchronized by external stimuli or zeitgebers, of which light is one of the most important, to the 24-hour solar cycle. When these zeitgebers are removed, as in experiments in bunkers, the biological clock will free-run and display its true circadian period which usually exceeds 24 hours. Rapid changes of shift, in contrast, will scramble the biological clock and reduce the amplitude and disrupt the phase of circadian rhythms.

We have previously shown that this can be done in nocturnal asthma when, on changing shifts, the rhythm in peak expiratory flow rate (PEFR) gradually re-establishes itself so that lowest PEFR is seen on waking, irrespective of the actual time of day. Patients vary in the speed at which they adjust, but in most of them this takes two to three days at least. Rapid shift changes will, therefore, obliterate the PEFR rhythm with reduction of its amplitude and reduce wheezing in association with the period of sleep (Hetzel and Clark 1980). This life-style is unacceptable to the average patient, however, and this approach has very little clinical value as a result.

Second, one can attempt to block the release or action of the various mediators which are believed to be responsible for nocturnal asthma. These might include the rhythmic secretion of cortisol, catecholamines, and histamine, and other mediators released by mast cells, together with changes in vagal tone. Thus corticosteroids, beta $_2$-stimulants, anticholinergic drugs, and sodium cromoglycate may all be relevant to this approach.

Finally, one can use drugs which might be expected to reduce bronchial lability or hyperreactivity. As discussed elsewhere in this volume, the nature of bronchial hyperreactivity is poorly understood, but sympathomimetic drugs, cromoglycate, and steroids may all be relevant here, since regular treatment with these agents has prophylactic value in reducing the severity of asthma.

To date, most research in the treatment of nocturnal asthma has related to beta$_2$stimulants in both aerosol and oral slow-release forms and to the methylxanthines. These are discussed in other sections of this volume and are clearly a logical first choice for study since they might be expected to compensate for the fall in circulating catecholamines at night, reduce mediator release from mast cells, and reduce bronchial lability. In this section I will discuss the relatively small amount of work which has been done on alternative drugs, with particular reference to sodium cromoglycate, corticosteroids, and anticholinergic drugs.

Sodium cromoglycate

Barnes *et al*. (1980) suggest that the rhythm in circulating catecholamines is a major factor in nocturnal asthma. At night they found a substantial rise in plasma histamine in asthmatics but very little change in normals. The nocturnal rise in histamine and fall in PEFR were reduced by low-dose infusions of adrenaline at night. They therefore postulate that falling catecholamine levels at night have a 'permissive' effect on mast cells with release of mediators and resulting bronchoconstriction. Whether inhibition of mast-cell degranulation is, in fact, responsible for the clinical efficacy of sodium cromoglycate has been questioned (Stokes and Morley 1981); since other drugs, more potent in inhibition of mast-cell degranulation in models such as the rat passive cutaneous anaphyllaxis test, have often shown no beneficial effect in subsequent clinical trials. Moreover, sympathomimetic drugs have been shown to be more potent than sodium cromoglycate in inhibition of histamine release from passively sensitized human chopped lung (Assem and Schild 1969). Nevertheless, sodium cromoglycate might be expected to be valuable in control of nocturnal asthma on the basis of nocturnal inhibition of mast-cell degranulation.

A further attraction of sodium cromoglycate is its low toxicity. The value of sympathomimetic drugs in nocturnal asthma may be more dependent on the magnitude of the dose than the choice of drug (Penketh *et al*. 1981). Control of nocturnal asthma may then only be achieved at the expense of unacceptable toxicity with tremor, restlessness, gastrointestinal disturbance, and other side-effects. Administration of sodium cromoglycate, however, might be effective in high doses in nocturnal asthma without toxicity. By giving high doses throughout the day, a beneficial effect in reducing bronchial lability might also be achieved.

The author's group have recently evaluated high-dose sodium cromoglycate in nocturnal asthma in a group of 20 patients (unpublished data). Patients were recruited who had overnight falls in PEFR of >25 per cent and nocturnal or early-morning wheezing. They kept diary charts of PEFR on waking, 1 hour after waking, at 16.00 hours, and at bedtime. They continued their usual treatment, including bronchodilator drugs, unchanged and monitored the number of extra doses of beta$_2$-stimulant aerosol required, in addition to regular treatment. Diary cards were kept for a two-week run-in period to ensure that patients satisfied our criteria of PEFR variation for entry into the trial and that they recorded data reliably. They then entered a double-blind cross-over study. In the first two weeks they inhaled a 2 ml vial in an electric nebuliser on waking, at 18.00 hours, and at bedtime and at lunch time they inhaled one capsule from a spinhaler. In the following two weeks they took 4 ml in the nebuliser and two spincaps at the same times. After a two-week washout they then took the other trial materials in the same doses in two further two-week periods. Treatments were with sodium cromoglycate or placebo. The low-dose active treatment was 80 mg sodium cromoglycate per day (20 mg as 2 ml of 1 per cent nebuliser solution x3 plus 20 mg by spincap) and the high-dose 280 mg daily (80 mg as 4 ml of 2 per cent nebuliser solution x3 plus 40 mg by spincaps).

At the time of writing, completed results are only available on nine patients who have completed the study. There were four males and five females. All were taking aerosol beta$_2$-stimulants and beclomethasone. Seven also took oral slow-release methylxanthines, four took oral corticosteroids, and two used slow-release oral salbutamol. One patient had episodes of flushing on treatment with cromoglycate, but no other side-effects were seen which could be definitely attributed to it.

Statistical analysis has not been carried out on this incomplete data but the available results suggest a trend of fewer nocturnal attacks and nights of disturbed sleep on the cromoglycate regimens when extra consumption of beta$_2$-aerosols also decreased. On placebo regimens there was no improvement in the mean overnight fall in PEFR from 15.9 per cent during the run-in or washout period to 15.6 per cent on both low- and high-dose placebo. On cromoglycate regimens the mean fall in PEFR during the run-in or washout period preceding treatment with cromoglycate was 12.9 per cent and reduced to 9.7 per cent on low-dose and 9.5 per cent on high-dose treatment.

Even if this apparent benefit is confirmed when data from the complete study is available, it is clear that the improvement with cromoglycate is small. Surprisingly there was no apparent relationship to the dose used with no increased benefit on the high-dose regimen. Rather similar results were obtained by Morgan *et al.* (1983) who gave a single nocturnal dose of 160 mg cromoglycate by nebulisation at bedtime in eight asthmatics. They were studied in hospital, in contrast to the author's out-patient study, and EEG and oxygen saturation were recorded during sleep. Response was compared with placebo in a double-blind cross-over study. There was no significant difference in the mean overnight fall in FEV$_1$ on placebo (from 2.5 to 1.8 L) compared with cromoglycate (from 2.4 to 1.9 L). The fall in FVC was significantly reduced by cromoglycate, but the improvement was small (3.8–3.0 L on placebo versus 3.9–3.23 L on cromoglycate). Oxygen saturation fell less on cromoglycate (5.7 per cent fall) overnight than on placebo (7.8 per cent). Less sleep disturbance and irregular breathing patterns were seen with cromoglycate.

Both these studies have shown some small benefit from cromoglycate, but this appears to consist predominantly in improved sleep rather than reduction in the overnight deterioration in lung function tests. High-dose cromoglycate was well tolerated but it is difficult to nebulise and the long time required to nebulise it is a problem for routine clinical use. These factors may partly account for the failure of higher doses of cromoglycate to produce further improvement in this study.

Ketotifen

This drug might be expected to be of value in nocturnal asthma on the rationale already discussed for cromoglycate. Different studies have, however, produced conflicting results for the clinical effectiveness of this drug (Lane 1980; Petheram *et al.* 1981). Monie *et al.* (1982) have provided some data on this question in a double-blind cross-over trial of ketotifen 1 mg b.d. versus cromoglycate 20 mg q.d.s. in a group of 28 asthmatics studied in two eight-week periods on each drug; both preceded by a two-week period on placebo. There was no overall benefit from ketotifen although there was improvement with cromoglycate. The overnight fall in PEFR was also investigated; although not the prime aim of the study. There was a significant improvement in the mean overnight fall in PEFR on placebo (43 L min^{-1}) on treatment with cromoglycate (25 L min^{-1}) but the fall on placebo before treatment with ketotifen (32 L min^{-1}) was not improved by ketotifen (50 L min^{-1}). The difference between results for cromoglycate and ketotifen was also significant. This study also, therefore, demonstrates a small benefit in nocturnal asthma from cromoglycate. One does occasionally come across patients who appear to have some improvement in nocturnal symptoms when treated with ketotifen but this could perhaps be due to the sedative effect of its antihistamine properties, rather than an effect on airway calibre.

Corticosteroids

It is difficult to assess the value of corticosteroids in nocturnal asthma in clinical practice since these drugs are very likely to have been included in the early treatment of more severe asthmatics, irrespective of whether they have nocturnal wheezing or not.

An early theory of the mechanism of nocturnal asthma was that it resulted from the fall in plasma cortisol at night and that the delayed action of corticosteroids in asthma explained the time lag between the lowest cortisol levels and lowest PEFR in the early hours of the morning. Abolition of the rhythm in plasma cortisol would be expected to prevent the nocturnal fall in PEFR if this were the case. Soutar *et al.* (1975) gave cortisol infusions to six asthmatics so that a constant cortisol level, in excess of the normal peak value of the circadian rhythm in plasma cortisol, was maintained throughout the 24-hour cycle. This had no effect on the rhythm in PEFR. Thus corticosteroids do not, apparently, prevent nocturnal asthma, but it should be noted that this study only considered a 24-hour period of treatment and did not look at the effects of continued steroid therapy.

Reinberg *et al.* (1974) studied the effects of a single dose of methylprednisolone in a group of six asthmatic boys at different times of day on different days. They found that the effect of steroids on improving mean daily PEFR was slightly affected by the time of day that treatment was given. Thus an improvement in mean PEFR of only four per cent was seen after treatment at 08.00 hours compared with 17 per cent on treatment at 15.00 hours. Moreover, treatment at 15.00 hours did alter the phase of the PEFR rhythm by delaying the acrophase (time of the peak reading of PEFR in the circadian cycle) from 14.00 hours before treatment to 20.00 hours after treatment. No benefit was seen, however, in the amplitude of the PEFR rhythm which increased from 25 per cent of the mean daily value to 28 per cent when treatment was given at 15.00 hours. Both these studies therefore show no effect of steroids in reducing the severity of nocturnal asthma.

Although controversy continues on the role of corticosteroids in acute asthma (Luska 1982; Grant 1982), most clinicians would agree that they play a major part in controlling severe acute asthma which has not responded to bronchodilator drugs and probably reduce mortality and the need for mechanical ventilation. The pattern of PEFR readings throughout the 24-hour cycle in some of these patients recovering from acute asthma does, however, suggest that corticosteroids can have a temporary adverse effect on nocturnal bronchoconstriction. Thus, as PEFR improves from the low levels seen on admission, the amplitude of PEFR variation starts to rise a day or two later and reaches a maximum, with increased nocturnal symptoms, a few days after admission. It is at this time that the risk of sudden death seems to be greatest in hospitalized patients (Hetzel *et al.* 1977). Subsequently, the amplitude of PEFR variation reduces somewhat as the patient returns to his usual PEFR levels when well. Steroids may, therefore, increase bronchial lability at these times and provoke increased nocturnal asthma. It is not clear, however, from these uncontrolled clinical observations, whether similar patterns would have been seen if these patients had not been given steroids. More data is needed on this question but, as with the treatment of acute asthma with steroids, controlled studies are not easily carried out in this situation.

It is easier to study the effects of inhaled steroids in nocturnal asthma since use of these drugs is more easily justified than the use of oral steroids in patients who have nocturnal wheezing but have near-normal lung function during the day and have not presented with acute asthma. Horn *et al.* (1984) studied 14 patients with nocturnal asthma. On initial treatment with inhaled salbutamol as rotacaps in a dose of 800 mcg four times a day, they achieved an improvement in mean PEFR of eight per cent and in eight cases there was a significant reduction in the 'morning dip' in PEFR to less than 50 per cent of the pretreatment value. Treatment was subsequently continued with the addition of becotide rotacaps 400 mcg q.d.s. There was a further improvement of five per cent in mean PEFR and eight cases now showed further reduction in the morning dip to <33 per cent of its original value with abolition of the dip in three of them. This study therefore provides some more objective evidence that steroids can reduce the amplitude of the PEFR rhythm and suggests that there is also an additive effect between beta$_2$-agonists and steroids. Before leaving the discussion of steroids in nocturnal asthma it is worth noting a further implication of the circadian rhythm in plasma cortisol in asthma which is that the suppressant effect of oral steroids on the hypothalamus–pituitary–adrenal axis is reduced by giving steroids in the morning, as opposed to divided doses during the day (McAllister *et al.* 1983).

Anticholinergic drugs

Anticholinergic drugs can reduce bronchoconstriction in asthma (Barber *et al.* 1977) but they are generally considered more useful in the treatment of airflow limitation associated with chronic bronchitis and emphysema (Crompton 1968). They are less popular in the treatment of young asthmatics where good response with no side-effects is usually seen on treatment with inhaled beta$_2$-agonists. There is some evidence that circadian variation in vagal tone may contribute to nocturnal asthma. Using sinus arrythmia gap as an indirect indicator of vagal tone, Soutar *et al.* (1977) showed some correlation between increased vagal activity at night and the fall in PEFR in asthma patients.

The synthetic anticholinergic drug ipratropium bromide is well tolerated by patients with airways obstruction and worthy of trial in nocturnal asthma. It is also safe in higher doses than those usually recommended i.e. 40 mg (Ruffin *et al.* 1978). Cox, Hughes, and McDonnell (unpublished data, personal communication) have recently studied the effects of a bedtime dose of 160 mcg ipratropium bromide. Fourteen patients with nocturnal asthma continued their usual therapy and were studied in open trial for three periods of two weeks. In the first two weeks they took their usual inhalation of 200 mcg salbutamol at bedtime. In the subsequent periods, in random order, they were given either 160 mcg ipratropium bromide alone or ipratropium bromide 160 mcg plus salbutamol 200 mcg. Mean overnight falls in PEFR were 242–191 L min^{-1} on salbutamol alone, 257–230 L min^{-1} on salbutamol plus ipratropium bromide, and 260–229 L min^{-1} on ipratropium bromide alone. Results for ipratropium bromide alone and in combination with salbutamol were significantly better than salbutamol alone. In addition to showing benefits from anticholinergic drugs in nocturnal asthma, this study suggests that ipratropium bromide may be superior to sulbutamol, but it must be remembered that a high dose of ipratropium bromide has been compared with a standard dose of salbutamol. High-dose inhalation therapy with salbutamol has also been shown to be effective in nocturnal asthma (Horn *et al*. 1984). Some patients in this study complained of dry mouth and two withdrew because of intolerance to the drug. Further studies of anticholinergic drugs are clearly indicated but they may prove to be less well tolerated than high-dose inhalation therapy with beta$_2$-agonists.

Bromocriptine

The dopaminergic agonist and prolactin inhibitor, bromocriptine, was evaluated in severe steroid-dependent asthmatics after it was noted that a patient treated with this drug for parkinsonism, who also had airways obstruction, became less wheezy during treatment. On this basis, Newman-Taylor *et al*. (1976) studied four severe asthmatics who also had nocturnal asthma. Treatment with bromocriptine in a dose of 20 mg daily resulted in improvement in three of them with reduction in both steroid requirements and nocturnal asthma. In one of these three, when bromocriptine was withdrawn because of side-effects, the nocturnal asthma recurred.

A subsequent study (Christensen *et al*. 1979) failed to confirm any benefit from bromocriptine. Twenty patients who were taking a mean dose of 10.7 mg prednisolone daily were studied in a controlled trial of 12-week treatment on both 15 mg daily of bromocriptine and placebo. This study showed no significant effect of bromocriptine on steroid requirements, consumption of bronchodilator drugs, or in diurnal variation in PEFR. On this evidence, there is little value in the use of this drug, which has a fairly high incidence of side-effects, in nocturnal asthma.

Naloxone

There has been recent interest in the role of the opioid peptides in asthma. They may mediate airways obstruction by acting as neurotransmitters in autonomic ganglia or by local hormonal effects. It has been shown that infusion of the encephalin analogue desamino metencephalin can precipitate asthma attacks (Leslie *et al*. 1980) and that the airways obstruction which can be induced in some diabetics by chlorpropamide and alcohol can be attenuated by prior administration of the specific opiate antagonist naloxone (Leslie *et al*. 1980). Since it has been shown that secretion of beta-endorphin has a circadian rhythm with peak levels betwen 04.00 and 10.00 hours (Dent *et al*. 1981), the effects of infusions of naloxone have been studied on the circadian rhythm in PEFR (Al-Damluji *et al*. 1983).

Six patients were recruited who had morning falls in PEFR of >25 per cent of the highest daily reading. They were studied over a 14-day period in a double-blind cross-over manner with infusions of naloxone on the fourth and fifth days and placebo on the ninth and tenth days; or vice versa. Infusions were given from 24.00 to 10.00 hours. Naloxone was given as a loading dose of 8 mg over 20 min, followed by 56 mg in 500 ml of saline at a rate of 5.6 mg/hour. There was no improvement in PEFR at 06.00 hours in comparison with placebo, and the only beneficial effect of naloxone was a small improvement in PEFR and FEV_1 between 08.00 and 20.00 hours but this was only seen after the first night's infusion. No very convincing reason was found for this observation, but the authors postulate that the nocturnal infusion of naloxone may have a delayed effect in improving airway calibre during the day and that administration of naloxone may have interfered with a negative feedback loop; thus provoking increased beta-encephalin secretion on the second day. In any event, these preliminary results do not suggest that the circadian rhythm in secretion of opiate peptides is likely to be an important factor in nocturnal asthma.

Conclusions

While many of these studies have been prompted by the limitations of $beta_2$-agonists and methylxanthines in the treatment of nocturnal asthma, these drugs remain the first line of treatment for this condition. Corticosteroids must also play a part in treatment as they are so often necessary in control of the patient's asthma, irrespective of nocturnal symptoms. More work is needed on their precise role in nocturnal asthma, however, and the possibility remains that they may temporarily provoke nocturnal wheezing in some patients recovering from acute asthma.

Of the other drugs considered, ipratropium bromide is clearly worthy of further study but may well prove less well tolerated than aerosol $beta_2$-stimulants. Sodium cromoglycate certainly has a slight beneficial effect but it is not yet clear whether this is dose-related and there are technical problems in giving higher doses in any case.

We clearly need new drugs for the treatment of nocturnal asthma since the application of existing agents to the problem is only partly effective. Development of the ideal treatment must clearly wait until the underlying mechanisms of nocturnal asthma are fully understood.

References

Al-Damluji, S., Thompson, P.J., Citron, K. and Turner-Warwick, M. (1983). *Thorax* **38**, 914.
Assem, E.S.K., and Schild, M.O. (1969). *Nature* **224**, 1028.
Barber, P.V., Chatterjee, S.S., and Scott, R. (1977). *Br. J. Dis. Chest* **71**, 101.
Barnes, P., Fitzgerald, G., Brown, M., and Dollery, C. (1980). *N. Engl. J. Med.* **303**, 263.
Christensen, K.M., Letman, H., and Mikkelsen, A.G. (1979). *Thorax* **34**, 284.
Crompton, G.R. (1968). *Thorax* **23**, 46.
Dent, R.N.M., Guillemenault, C., Albert, L.H., Posner, B.I., Cox, B.M., and Goldstein, A. (1981). *J. clin. Endocrinol. Metab.* **52**, 942.
Grant, I.W.B. (1982). *Br. J. Dis. Chest* **26**, 125.
Hetzel, M.R. and Clark, T.J.H. (1980). In *Chronopharmacology* (ed. A. Reinberg and F. Halberg), p.213. Pergamon, Oxford.
Hetzel, M.R., Clark, T.J.H., and Branthwaite, M.A. (1977). *Br. med. J.* **1**, 808.
Horn, C.R., Clark, T.J.H., and Cochrane, G.M. (1984). *Thorax* **39**, (in press).
Lane, D.J. (1980). *Clin. Allergy* **10**, 519.
Leslie, R.D.G., Bellamy, D., and Pyke, D.A. (1980). *Br. med. J.* **1**, 16.
Luska, A.R. (1982). *Br. J. Dis. Chest* **76**, 15.
McAllister, W.A.C., Hetzel, M.R., Emery, P., Gotham, C.R., and Collins, J.V. (1983). *Thorax* **38**, 230.
Monie, R.D., Peter-Smith, A., Leopold, D., Anderson, G., Davies, B.H., and Thomas, G.J. (1982). *Br. J. Dis. Chest* **76**, 383.

Morgan, A.D., Connaughton, J.J., Catterall, J.R., Shapiro, C.M., Douglas, N.J., and Flenley, D.C. (1983). *Proc. Med. Res. Soc.* p.7p.
Newman-Taylor, A.J., Soutar, C., Schneerson, J., and Turner-Warwick, M. (1976). *Thorax* **31**, 488.
Penketh, A.R.L., Johnson, D., Hetzel, M.R., Clark, T.J.H., Bellamy, D., and Cochrane, G.M. (1981). *Thorax* **36**, 715.
Petheram, I.S., Moxham, J., Bierman, C.W., Mc Allen, M., Spiro, S.G. (1981). *Thorax* **36**, 308.
Reinberg, A., Halberg, F., and Falliers, C.J. (1974). *Chronobiologica* **1**, 333.
Ruffin, R.E., Wolf, R.K., Dolovich, M.B., Rossman, C.M., and Fitzgerald, J.D. (1978). *Chest* **73**, 501.
Soutar, C.A., Carruthers, M., and Pickering, C.A. (1977). *Thorax* **32**, 677.
Soutar, C.A., Costello, J., Ijaduola, O., and Turner-Warwick, M. (1975). *Thorax* **30**, 436.
Stokes, T.C., and Morley, J. (1981). *Br. J. Dis. Chest* **75**, 1.
Willis, T. (1679). *Pharmaceutice rationalis*, Vol. 2. Dring, Harper, Leigh, London.

Summary of treatment

D.C. FLENLEY

Department of Respiratory Medicine, University of Edinburgh, City Hospital, Edinburgh, UK.

What have we learned in terms of understanding nocturnal asthma? I think the answer is that there is a great deal yet to do, in the hope that better understanding of mechanisms will improve treatment — or prevention.

In discussing the treatment it is important also to enquire how the drugs affect the patients' sleep, but this aspect seems so far to have been largely neglected. I find it difficult to believe that someone who is so poisoned with a β_2-agonist that the bed is shaking is having an adequate night's sleep. In future studies it will be important to assess not only peak flow in the morning but also how the patient has slept. Professor Turner-Warwick showed how common the symptom of nocturnal or early morning wheeze is, but usually if you ask an asthmatic about how he slept the answer is 'fine', because that is a social question. But if you ask how often they wake at night wheezy and breathless, the answer often is 'Doesn't everybody wake at night wheezy and breathless?' This is an extremely common symptom if you ask about it, and something needs to be done to relieve it.

Asthma affects four to ten per cent of children. I don't think that they are going to perform very well in school if they have been up wheezing all the night previously, so that we can potentially make a very important contribution if we could improve this symptom. We have heard that β_2-agonists have a problem as they don't last long enough if given by the preferred route, which is by inhalation, although there is some suggestion from recent work that bigger doses might prolong the effect, and I think that needs to be confirmed in larger numbers of subjects. Giving large doses of β_2-agonists by mouth is not particularly effective, but does cause side-effects, and I suggest that you may not sleep very well if you have tremor, tachycardia, and anxiety.

We have heard that slow-release theophyllines are effective at night. However, there is enormous variability in the plasma level achieved by chronic administration of standard oral doses of these drugs, and it is important to know the serum levels if theophyllines are to be used properly. In Dr Fairfax's study the serum levels of theophylline were not high enough to be able to say that the patient was getting effective therapy. Is there a place for interaction between β_2-agonists and theophyllines? Svedmyr and Svedmyr (1982) have shown that you can achieve a trade-off by using β_2-agonist by inhalation, combined with a therapeutic level of serum theophylline from an oral dose, so as to get an additive bronchodilator effect, without the addition of side-effects.

The effect of oral steroids is difficult to evaluate. Oscillations in peak flow increase in amplitude as the patient recovers from an acute attack, in patients who have had oral steroids. Fanta *et al.* (1983) have now clearly shown that steroids speed the recovery from acute severe asthma. Steroids probably do also have a place in management of nocturnal asthma, but there is need to define their role more precisely.

As far as the other drugs which were briefly referred to, I agree entirely with what was said about cromoglycate in preventing nocturnal wheeze: it was a nice idea but it doesn't work particularly well. Ketotifen, as our own studies have shown (Catterall *et al.* 1983) is a good hypnotic in asthma and that brings me to sedatives. Most asthmatics are looked after by their own GPs and, if an asthmatic says he doesn't sleep very well, I suspect he may often be given a hypnotic such as a benzodiazepine. It would be nice to know how commonly this occurs, and what effects it may have. Surprisingly the most common tablet taken in the UK to help sleep may well be aspirin, and we do not know if this will have any effect on nocturnal asthma, even in those patients who do not have aspirin-induced asthma.

This book has indicated controversial areas, where we disagree. The answer to scientific disagreement is to design better studies, and more studies are clearly needed in nocturnal asthma. As far as treatment is concerned I suggest that if you have a patient with nocturnal asthma, who doesn't warrant oral steroids, it is reasonable to start with inhaled β_2-agonists with slow-release theophylline by mouth, both given on retiring, as I do not think that inhaled β_2-agonist alone will last long enough throughout the night. If the patient is not much better in a week, then the therapy can be escalated. I think that we still need better and longer-acting drugs, but as well as measuring the peak expiratory flow rate in the morning, we should also have more information on how the patients actually sleep.

References

Catterall, J.R., Calverley, P.M.A., Power, J.T., Shapiro, C.M., Douglas, N.J. and Flenley, D.C. (1983). *Thorax* **38**, 845.
Fanta, C.H., Rossing, T.J., and McFadden, E.R. (1983). *Am. J. Med.* **74**, 845.
Hockley, B., Johnson, N., and McKay, (1983). *Postgrad. med. J.* **59**, 504.
Svedmyr, K. and Svedmyr, N. (1982). *Allergy* **37**, 101.